Penny Gulliver's Self-Defence Handbook for Women

*To my mother, Pauline;
my father, Barry; and my
grandmother, Olga*

Penny Gulliver's Self-Defence Handbook for Women

Hale & Iremonger

DISCLAIMER

All care has been taken to ensure that the information contained in this book has been presented in a responsible manner and is not dangerous or harmful but no responsibility is accepted for any errors or omissions. The Authors and the Publisher on its own behalf and that of its employees agents consultants and advisers disclaim liability for all loss, damage or injury, financial or otherwise, suffered by any person acting upon or relying on the information and advice in this book, whether resulting from the negligence of the Authors or the Publisher or its employees agents consultants or advisers or from any other cause whatsoever.

© 1994 by Penny Gulliver

This book is copyright. Apart from any fair dealing for the purposes of study, research, criticism, review, or as otherwise permitted under the Copyright Act, no part may be reproduced by any process without written permission. Inquiries should be made to the publisher.

Typeset, printed & bound by
Southwood Press Pty Limited
80–92 Chapel Street, Marrickville, NSW

For the publisher
Hale & Iremonger Pty Limited
GPO Box 2552, Sydney, NSW

National Library of Australia Cataloguing-in-publication entry

Gulliver, Penny, 1955- .

    Penny Gulliver's self-defence handbook for women.

    Bibliography.

    ISBN 0 86806 497 1.

    1. Self-defence for women. I. Title. II. Title: Self-defence handbook for women.

613.66082

Front cover photograph: C. Moore Hardy.
Back cover photographs: C. Moore Hardy and Aref, courtesy of *Looks Magazine*.
Photographs throughout: C. Moore Hardy, the author, *Woman's Day*, and contributions courtesy of Sandy Edwards and Terry Lee.

Contents

	Introduction	7
1	Sugar and spice: Tactics for survival	9
2	Bread and butter: Basic strikes	22
3	Attacks from the front	42
4	Attacks from behind	50
5	Down, but not out: Fighting back from the ground	59
6	Blocking techniques for punches and weapons	69
7	Machismo: Is there a cure?	85
8	Domestic violence	94
9	What to do if you are raped	98
10	Psychological self-defence: Prevention is better than cure	111
11	Women with special needs	121
12	The martial arts: Which one?	137
	Appendix Warming up	151
	Bibliography	156
	Acknowledgements	159

I might be small and still shy but I don't think I would panic now . . . [Penny Gulliver's course] has given me enormous confidence, all women should be taught this.

— A former student

I would highly recommend Penny's course to anyone. It is a fun way to learn important practical skills. The course empowers women and raises their confidence and self-esteem, provides motivation and offers a range of solutions to many situations. It takes away the fear of being helpless or a victim. The workplace aspects of women at risk was particularly enlightening, in this respect the course should be a compulsory part of every woman's personal development and safety training.

— Lynne Black
Business Services Officer
Water Board, Sydney-Illawarra-Blue Mountains

This is a long overdue letter to thank you very much for teaching me the self-defence skills I learnt two or so years ago . . . I was mugged at Circular Quay one evening. The man approached me from behind, and I was quick thinking enough to give him a very sore groin and shins! I had always imagined I would freeze in such a situation, but I didn't. So thank you, I got away!

— Julia Forsyth
A former student

Introduction

This book contains the seeds of empowerment. If they are planted in the soil of commitment to personal safety and nurtured on determination and fearless resolve, they have the potential to bear the fruits of self-esteem, cunning, and resourcefulness.

I want to inspire every reader to make this deep commitment to personal safety, because without this inspiration there will be no perspiration. Thus the three levels of this book are: to inspire; to instruct; and to entertain.

This book examines how women see themselves and considers how our self-perceptions effect the ways we respond to danger and the need for self-protection. Since a woman's effectiveness in an assault will depend primarily on how she feels about herself (her worth, her rights and her powerfulness) and on how much she is prepared to act on these feelings, this book and many of its exercises will focus upon these feelings and responses.

As you read this book remember that it is not enough to simply learn the self-defence techniques — learning to paint-by-numbers won't turn you into Leonardo da Vinci. As well you will require a creative, positive approach and some application (that is, practice) in order to develop your basic and essential survival skills.

The first thing to realise is that feeling afraid is not bad. If someone attacks us we naturally will feel afraid, just like anybody else, and that feeling is useful because it ensures that we react. We must use our fear, channel it, and transform it into a positive energy that works for us, not against us. We must tap our survival instinct. It, unlike the fairy tale rescuer, Prince Charming, can always be counted on to appear when it is most desperately needed.

It's always with us waiting to serve us. We can rely upon it to be there when we need it most. Which is more than we can say for Prince Charming. He might not be conveniently at hand or, if he is, he may possibly not feel inclined to risk his neck in order to save ours.

Being attacked will be the loneliest moment of your life. To prepare for that moment and to help prevent it from arriving, it's very important that you cultivate a sense of independence, of physical and emotional resourcefulness. It is important to see that there are untapped parts of you that are strong, valiant, brave, courageous, fearless, heroic, capable, independent, assertive, determined, instinctive and, if the situation calls for it, ruthless. These qualities constitute what I call 'the warrior spirit'. These are the qualities we look for and expect to find in our Prince Charming. Our power increases when these 'masculine' qualities are balanced with what I call the Snow White qualities. These are the 'feminine' qualities of intuition, perception, persuasion and cunning. Women must cultivate a wide range of emotional expression, so that when the situation calls for it they can be tough.

Unfortunately, due to our social conditioning and to the roles convention assigns to us – me Tarzan, you Jane – we are polarised by our gender differences. Let's try and break through these barriers. At best, stereotypes cripple our ability to be a whole person, and, at worst, they prevent us from defending ourselves.

The exercises given in each chapter will challenge you physically and emotionally. They may be worked through consecutively or randomly, but only when you have covered all the material will you get a complete picture of the diverse strategies available to you.

I don't have the patent on survival strategies. Every woman has the ability to develop her own tactics. Take an active and creative approach to your personal safety and to the reading of this book.

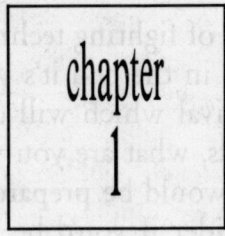

Sugar and spice:
Tactics for survival

As little girls growing up we were told that we were supposed to be 'sugar and spice and all things nice', as opposed to 'slugs and snails and puppy dogs' tails' (the male counterpart). Both alternatives strike me as distinctly unattractive. If we live up to our prescribed role, which most of us count on for our validation, we in fact restrict our capabilities to deal with an attack, not to mention every other area of our life! We must uproot our sense of ourselves from this infertile soil, transplant it and nurture a new creative, dynamic self-definition, so that we can feel OK, even when we are not 'nice': because ninety-eight per cent of the time being 'nice' will not save us from being raped, murdered or harassed. How can we do this? Here is a kaleidoscope of strategies and characteristics that are interdependent and effective:

Versatility
Having as many tricks up our sleeves as possible is the first step to safety.

Self-esteem
It's hard to fight off or discourage a potential assailant if we don't feel we are worth fighting for! About ninety per cent of our communication with other people is conveyed by our body language and tone of voice, so if we don't accept our inner selves, it usually shows. We must take a long hard look at what we have been taught makes us feel good about ourselves as women, and at the images we learn we must live up to in order to gain approval.

Commitment

You can learn thousands of fighting techniques and study martial arts for many years, but in the end it's your emotional commitment to your own survival which will determine how safe you really are. In other words, what are you willing to do to survive? Ask yourself what you would be prepared to do to protect your children, and then consider if you'd be prepared to go to those same lengths to protect yourself. If you are like most of us — professional, unpaid, taken-for-granted caregivers — your answer will probably indicate that you would be much more ruthless in the defence of your children than you would be in your own self-defence.

True commitment to our survival means that we are willing to fight for our freedom and our lives, as well as for that of our families. We're prepared to fight, and fight dirty, not with the Marquis of Queensberry's rules! Squeamishness has no place when you are fighting for your life.

Here is a checklist on ruthlessness to see if you are prepared to strike and strike HARD at the vulnerable areas of an attacker's body. Would you be prepared to:
- Bite the top lip or nose of an assailant if you were pinned down? (This can send the attacker into shock.)
- Squash an exposed scrotum?
- Jab a pen or sharp object at the throat of an attacker?
- Scratch the corneas of the eyes with your fingernails?

These tactics indeed show 'no mercy', but how much mercy do you think you will get from your attacker? Mercy is a luxury we sometimes cannot afford. If it has to be them or us, let it be the attacker! This is not to say that if some drunk gets a bit 'touchy-feely' at a party that we must bite his top lip off (even if you might feel like it)! In Chapter 10 we will deal with appropriate assertiveness techniques for such occasions.

You must gear your response to the level of muscle that the circumstances may warrant. We must keep reaffirming our new definition of self-esteem and self-love, enmeshing it with our right to choose who touches our bodies and how we have them touched. After all, this is no more than our individual right to control our physical, mental and spiritual destiny, because, if one of those

SUGAR AND SPICE: TACTICS FOR SURVIVAL

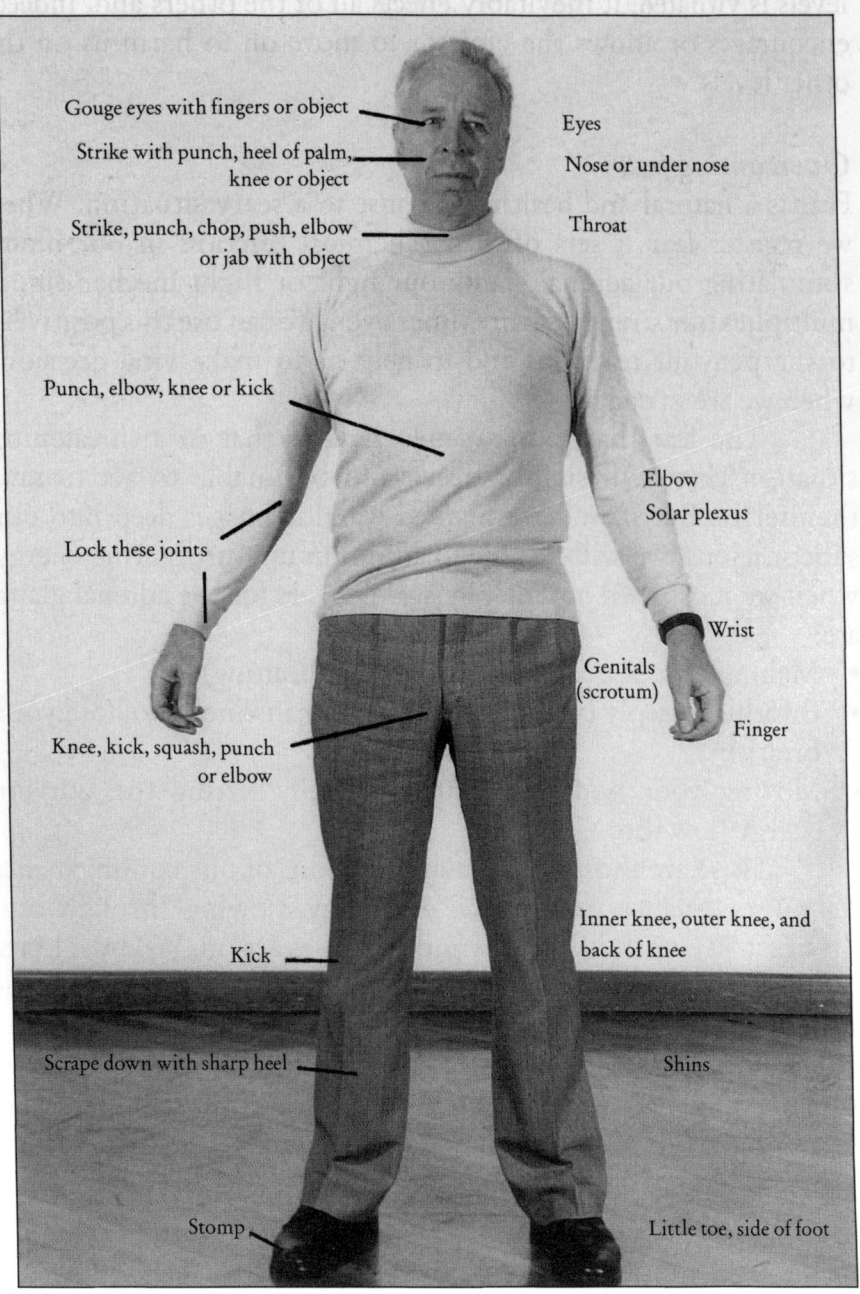

STRIKES   **VULNERABLE POINTS**

levels is violated, it inevitably effects all of the others and, indeed, encourages or allows the violator to move on to harm us on the other levels.

Overcoming fear

Fear is a natural and healthy response to a scary situation. When we register fear it sets off a biochemical reaction in our brain, stimulating our adrenal gland: our fight or flight mechanism. It multiplies our strength many times over. We can use this positively to sharpen our reactions and to help us to make vital decisions when we are in danger.

The fear that most women have is that in a threatening situation they will simply freeze and be unable to act to save themselves. But if we have planted warrior images deep into our subconscious, we will be able to summon up our fighting energy when we most need it. The physical triggers for the adrenal gland are:

- Making a lot of noise (e.g. screaming, shouting);
- Breathing deeply (when you freeze your instinct is to hold your breath);
- Moving your body vigorously, thereby letting the warrior energy flow through you.

These are the physical manifestations of our commitment. We must visualise our source of energy, flowing through our physical and emotional blocks and issuing as action. We must learn to appreciate our fear as a stimulus for adrenalin, energy, movement, and courage.

This courage will enable us to take responsibility for our own safety and defence. If we confront our fears on this level the world will be our oyster. We'll find that many other situations that have evoked fear will be challenged, so that we can go deeper into every area of our lives.

Energy

Energy is your source of life. It is the fuel you put into your tank of techniques. If you put no fuel in your engine, you are not going to move anywhere. The energies used to fuel the techniques covered in this book can be linked to the four basic elements – Fire, Earth, Water and Air. Once you have grasped a basic understanding of how these techniques develop all of these energies, I encourage you to go off and devise and discover your own style of movement and

SUGAR AND SPICE: TACTICS FOR SURVIVAL

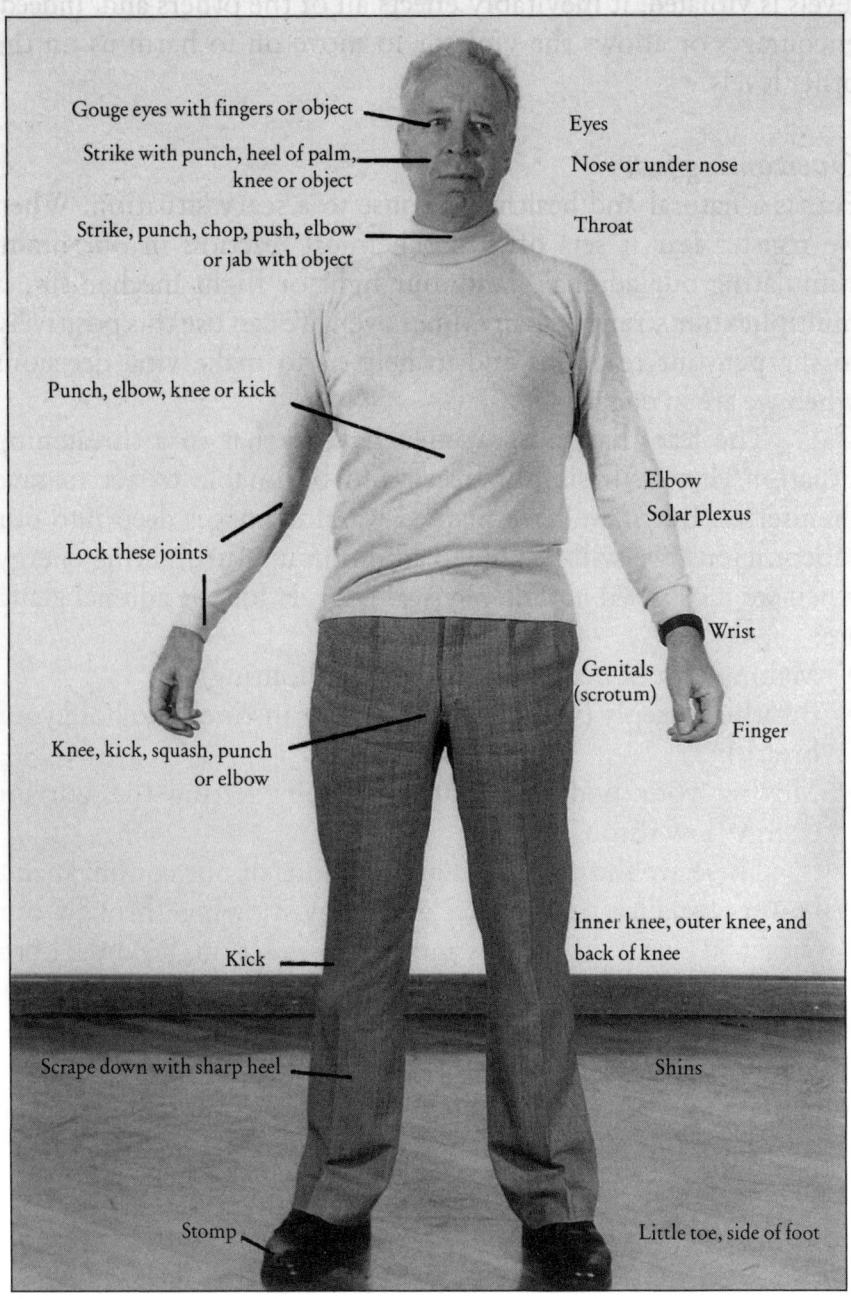

STRIKES   **VULNERABLE POINTS**

levels is violated, it inevitably effects all of the others and, indeed, encourages or allows the violator to move on to harm us on the other levels.

Overcoming fear
Fear is a natural and healthy response to a scary situation. When we register fear it sets off a biochemical reaction in our brain, stimulating our adrenal gland: our fight or flight mechanism. It multiplies our strength many times over. We can use this positively to sharpen our reactions and to help us to make vital decisions when we are in danger.

The fear that most women have is that in a threatening situation they will simply freeze and be unable to act to save themselves. But if we have planted warrior images deep into our subconscious, we will be able to summon up our fighting energy when we most need it. The physical triggers for the adrenal gland are:

- Making a lot of noise (e.g. screaming, shouting);
- Breathing deeply (when you freeze your instinct is to hold your breath);
- Moving your body vigorously, thereby letting the warrior energy flow through you.

These are the physical manifestations of our commitment. We must visualise our source of energy, flowing through our physical and emotional blocks and issuing as action. We must learn to appreciate our fear as a stimulus for adrenalin, energy, movement, and courage.

This courage will enable us to take responsibility for our own safety and defence. If we confront our fears on this level the world will be our oyster. We'll find that many other situations that have evoked fear will be challenged, so that we can go deeper into every area of our lives.

Energy
Energy is your source of life. It is the fuel you put into your tank of techniques. If you put no fuel in your engine, you are not going to move anywhere. The energies used to fuel the techniques covered in this book can be linked to the four basic elements – Fire, Earth, Water and Air. Once you have grasped a basic understanding of how these techniques develop all of these energies, I encourage you to go off and devise and discover your own style of movement and

flow. In traditional martial arts this dance of movements, of one movement flowing out of another, often flowing from one energy source to another is called kata or forms. Let's look at the four elemental energy sources (here I am indebted to Kaleghl Quinn's *A Woman's Guide to Self-Preservation: Stand Your Ground*, London, Macdonald Optima, 1983, for her inspiration):

Fire This is the most useful element. Rising from the lower abdomen, it burns rapidly throughout your body giving you agility and speed and enabling you to strike and evade noisily and explosively.

Earth This is your grounding. Connection with the earth, usually with your feet, gives you stability, helping you to keep your stance and balance when someone is trying to unbalance you. Here lies your centredness and solidity. Once grounded on earth, practical thinking under stress becomes possible. Hard and strong punching makes the ground your friend.

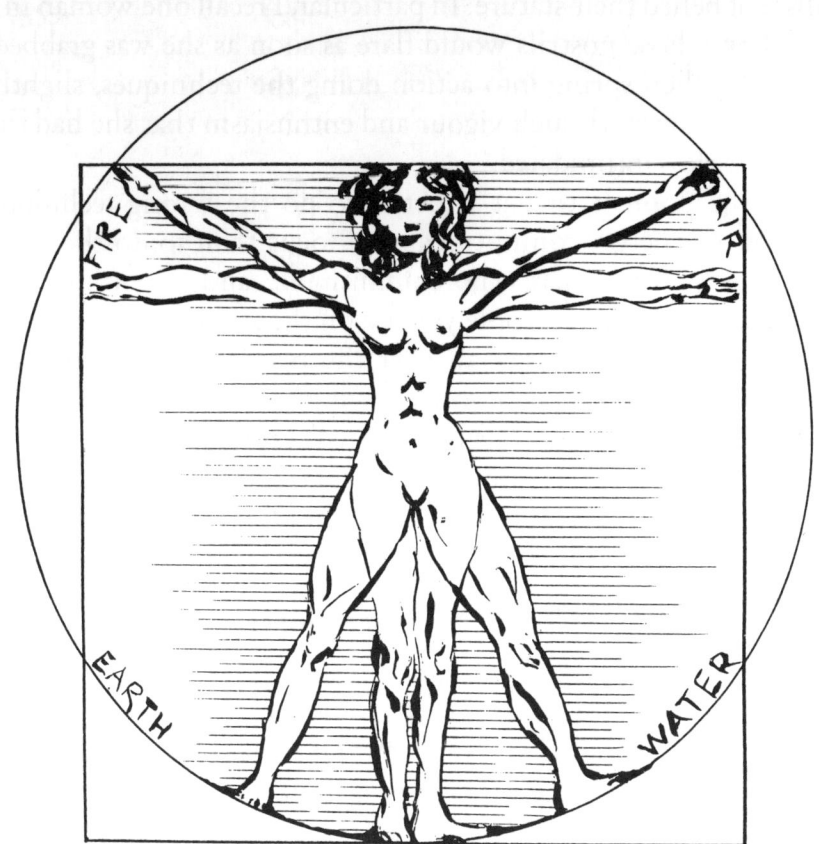

Water This enables you to blend with an opposing force. When someone is trying to punch you, you go with their energy, using it against them. This type of energy uses intuition, instinct, circular movement, fluidity, softness, and flexibility, using it enables you to fall and roll with the punches.

Air This is the intangible. When the attacker attacks, you aren't there. Elusive, evasive, invisible, if someone tries to strike you with a knife all they get is the air, because you aren't there. (The trick is to maintain your distance, and when the attacker moves forward, you move back, keeping the air between you.)

These concepts will help you to start to feel and not just think about how to act and react in a threatening situation.

Energy does not necessarily rely on physical strength and scientific analysis. It can be explained as a force field or it may be expressed as a dance. Energy allows us to transcend our size and muscular limitations. Indeed, I have found many diminutive women to have astounding warrior energy and self-preservation skills that belied their stature. In particular, I recall one woman in a workshop whose nostrils would flare as soon as she was grabbed. She would then spring into action doing the techniques, slightly incorrectly, but with such vigour and enthusiasm that she had the rest of the class intimidated.

The point is that it is better to do the wrong technique with lots of energy, commitment and focus than to do the right technique with no energy, no commitment, and no enthusiasm. For instance, consider people you see on the street who are out of control, with their energy all over the place. They are usually mentally disturbed, and beyond bowing to sex-role stereotypes. Their energy is usually erratic, unpredictable, uninhibited and usually they have four times the strength of a normal person. They feel very little fear and feel less pain. You could consciously imitate that behaviour if you found yourself in a tight spot – an attacker would think twice about attacking someone he suspected might lose control.

A series of techniques can be used quickly and smoothly in a creative and effective way as the energy flows through the body and out towards the assailant, who receives a barrage of energy flowing in rapid unrelenting succession and directed towards striking, breaking holds, rolling, distracting and moving out of the situation. Rather than thinking of escape techniques individually and in isolation from each other, employ creativity, versatility, mobility, originality and adaptability to give you dynamic ways to ensure your survival.

Intuition

Knowing without proof is a virtue for which women have long been admired. Intuition is definitely a quality we must value and use. It can warn us to refuse lifts with friends or strangers when we get a funny feeling about them and their intentions; it can urge us to walk in a different direction home from shopping, because we feel odd about someone in the vicinity; or get us to cancel a date with someone because of the vibes he sends.

One of my students had just met a fellow at a night club in Sydney and liked him initially. He asked her to go to a party on the other side of town. She had agreed to go with him until he started 'jokingly' grabbing her from behind with his arm around her neck, playing mock attack games. She decided these displays of dominance were not good signs of what was to come, so she cancelled the date. So, if your intuition warns you that something is wrong:

- Keep two arms' length away from anyone who tries to come unwelcomed into your personal space;
- Ask a friend to come and stay with you if you are at home alone and you get a funny feeling that there is someone outside your house;
- Leave a situation (party, house, office, car) where you sense a problem.

Observe early warning signs

The physical manifestations of intuition should be used as your in-built barometer of trouble. It may be a pain in the stomach, a sinking sensation in the knees, giddiness or any one of a host of physical symptoms. It's important to discover what your own personal body's wariness reaction may be and not to deny the signals or funny feelings your body is sending you. So many women experience these feelings and then ignore them. We have to learn to trust ourselves and our judgment.

Write down your early warning signs. What are they? Write down a list of times when you have experienced these. What has happened?

Surprise

The element of surprise can be simultaneously our best friend and our worst enemy. The good news is that most attackers see themselves as hunters after prey and they are not expecting a high level of effective resistance. Just remember that most attackers are known to their victim and may be under the misapprehension that a woman is playing hard to get: 'I'm sure she wants it, she's just playing games'. Even strangers may deceive themselves in this way or they may simply objectify and dehumanise the object of their attack, so that they don't consider that their victim has any feelings at all.

Some men may think rape is a man's right: 'If a woman doesn't want to give it, the man should take it. Women have no right to say no. Women are made to have sex. It's all they're good for. Some women would prefer to take a beating, but they always give in. It's what they are for'. (From an interview with an imprisoned rapist, quoted in Bart & O'Brien, *Stopping Rape: Successful Survival Strategies*, Oxford, Pergamon, 1985, p. 100.)

We must counter expectations of submission and ineffectiveness with a few little surprises of our own, such as commitment to self-determination, explosiveness, effectiveness and ruthlessness, if necessary. We must use all the strategies at our disposal. A woman willing to fight back effectively will come as a big shock to most men.

The bad news is that, if we haven't heeded our early warning signs or are caught totally unprepared, it's much harder to combat an assailant.

Distraction

This is closely linked to the element of surprise. Most attackers are going to be bigger and stronger than the women that they are attacking. Our ability to distract may be defined as the way we can stop this larger and stronger force from being directed towards us and deflect it onto something else, even if momentarily, in order to give us the chance to escape.

Distractions may be divided into a number of categories:

i. *Pain* If an attacker feels sharp pain or finds himself unable to breathe, this can lessen his commitment to his intended aim. It's important that the pain is sufficient to stop him in his tracks rather than just annoy him which might have the effect of simply aggravating the situation.

Strike vulnerable areas of your attacker with your own body (Chapter 2) or with an object from your environment – a chair, lamp, pen, etc. (In these situations it's better not to hesitate or threaten, because the weapon can be taken from you.)

ii. *Talking* You may be able to talk an assailant out of his intention. Some approaches that have proved effective include getting the rapist to identify with your humanity: 'How would you feel if this were happening to your sister, daughter, mother?' Tune into your intuition to see what you can detect about the attacker's emotions and areas of vulnerability. One woman talked her attacker down by saying, 'You look like nobody has ever listened to you'. The woman then proceeded to counsel her attacker, thus redirecting his energies into dealing with his emotions.

Claiming to have an infectious and dangerous disease such as AIDS, herpes, or VD has also proven effective in dissuading a would-be rapist.

Once he feels he has you, the attacker could be open to bargaining. For instance: 'I tried using as much naivete as I could ... I told him that I was really frightened of getting pregnant, that I would have to tell my mother if I was pregnant and my boyfriend. He said, "It's all right honey we aren't going to make any babies tonight," and then he withdrew before ejaculation.' (Bart & O'Brien, p. 54.)

A distinction needs to be drawn between talking your way out of a situation and pleading or begging. Beseeching has been shown to be a pretty useless tactic because it reaffirms your position as the victim, the very position that your attacker desires to put you in. Pleading doesn't act as a deterrent at all, rather it often encourages the situation to develop. Generally, talking your way out of a situation has proven less effective than actively fighting back with commitment and intention.

iii. *Cunning* There may be some situations where it is virtually impossible to get away. For instance, the attacker may have started sexually assaulting his victim. In some cases this may be the best time to act because the attacker is probably distracted by what he is doing. The movie 'Extremities', starring Farrah Fawcett, shows the attacker fondling his victim. She has been unable to get away. He moves down her body caressing and fondling her mid-section. He is not watching what she is doing with her arms. She grabs a can of pesticide, squirts it in his eyes and then hits him over the head with a saucepan, ties him up, and shoves him in the fireplace. The assailant in the movie has already raped and murdered two women, yet appears to lead a respectable life as a husband and father. The point to be made here is that a man is more likely to kill his victim after he's raped her.

Another excellent example of distraction may be illustrated in 'The Deer-Hunter'. Robert De Niro and friend have been captured by the Viet Cong and must play a game of Russian Roulette to avoid a slower, more painful death. Robert De Niro distracts his captors by getting them all laughing, then he and his friend grab two of the six machine-guns that have been pointed at both of them and manage to escape. (This is the story I tell my younger students who always seem to then ask impossible questions like, 'What if they have six machine-guns pointed at your head?' Remember nothing is impossible!)

iv. *Loud noise* When we were small children loud noise was one of our fears. This fear remains with us as adults and can be used as a primary distraction tool. The noise may be either your own screams and yells, or it can come from something breaking, or even from an external coincidental noise over which you have no control. I have been told of several incidents where a car back-firing, a window breaking, a TV set thrown down and exploding, or a siren happening to sound in the vicinity have each been sufficient to make an attacker flee. Distraction can be creative. You never know what might work. Perhaps bizarre behaviour, such as pulling faces or other inappropriate actions may be distracting and unsettling enough to an attacker to momentarily loosen his grip or divert him long enough for you to kick him swiftly in the groin.

One woman who was attacked by a man in a balaclava managed to escape once she was already pinned down on the ground. She told her attacker that she was having her period and she had to 'fix herself up'. He raised up off her just enough so she could kick him in the groin with enough power to propel him across the room.

v. *External intervention* Seeking and accepting outside help is very important. It's much better to get someone to help you than to deal with the situation alone.

Don't misinterpret this statement to mean that you don't need to develop your own resources to their optimum. You do. What I mean is, that if you don't have to put yourself at risk by fighting someone off, then don't. Part of your survival technique should be to attract the attention of someone who can help you, particularly the authorities.

Many women have told me that they get no response from just screaming, as many people don't take this seriously or don't want to get involved and place themselves at risk. It has been suggested that victims yell 'Fire' instead of 'Help', since it's more likely to attract attention. There may be some kind of code system you can develop within your community so that a certain word shouted loudly can mean someone is in trouble.

vi. *Using your environment* If you are in your own home take advantage of the fact that you know your way around and the attacker doesn't. Always assess the exit points for a potential escape route. Remember that anything and everything can be brandished as a weapon if you don't want to strike the attacker with your fist or foot. You may use dirt from a pot plant to throw in their eyes, or you could break the television or a window in order to attract attention and possibly external intervention, as well as quite likely alarming your attacker. It's wise once your early warning signs have started to tingle to start assessing potential weapons, escape routes and rescuers who could intervene between you and the attacker.

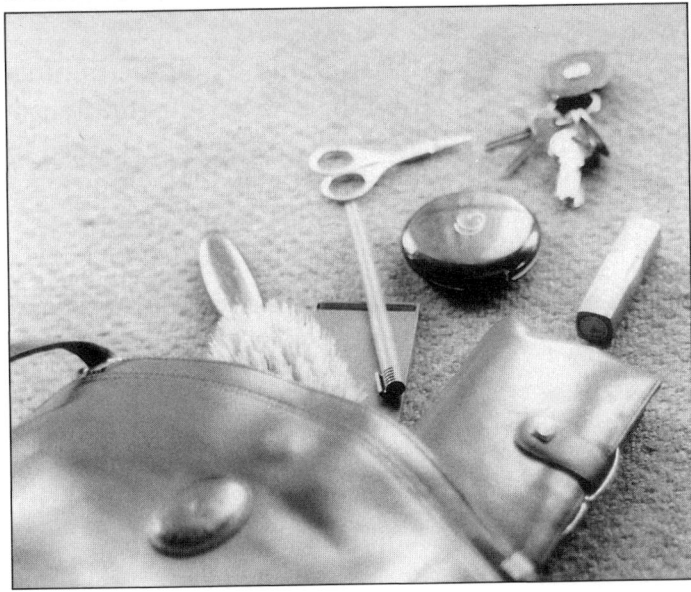

Typical handbag arsenal

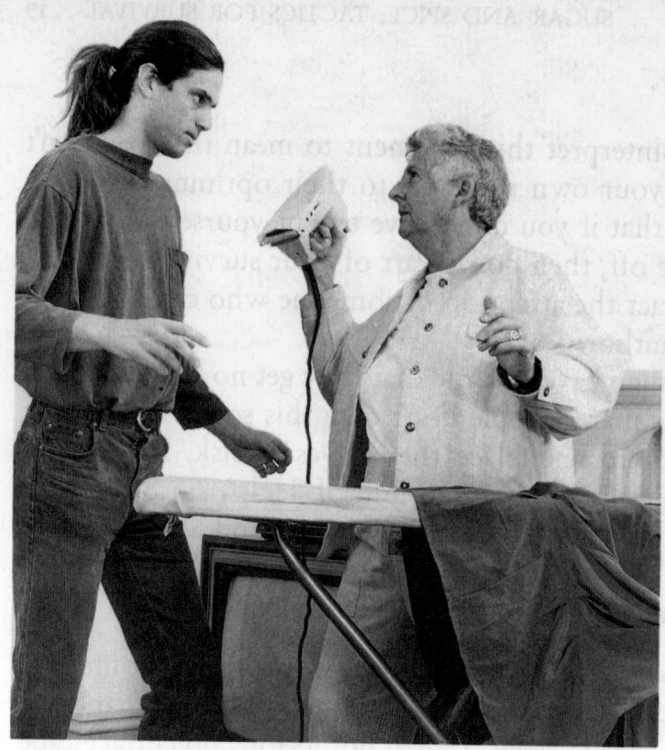

'Back-off' using available weapon

A list of potential weapons might include keys wedged between your fingers, a nail-file, an alarm, an umbrella, scissors, a comb, a hatpin, spray perfume, rolled-up newspaper, and any heavy object that can be used as a missile or club. You could be carrying a veritable arsenal in your handbag.

Men are often afraid of male authority, so when possible threaten to attract the attention of someone who seems to have authority (for instance, someone in a uniform — a security guard, bus driver, police officer).

Once when I was living in a flat in Bondi, I heard screaming from next-door. The woman who lived there was being threatened with a knife by her drunken boyfriend. I went in. First I asked if she wanted some help. She said she did, so I stood between them and looked him straight in the eye and told him I would ring the police if he didn't leave, at which point he retreated slowly, shouting obscenities as he went. The threat of a uniform was enough to deter him.

vii. *Fleeing* This is a fairly obvious and highly successful strategy. The best thing you can do if you sense danger is to leave or run away. In one case recounted in *Stopping Rape*, a man approached a woman from behind and held a sharp object to her back, saying that she would be alright if she didn't try to put up a fight. Instead, she fled immediately upon being attacked and thereby avoided being raped. (Bart & O'Brien, p. 43.)

Conclusion

No specific martial art has the patent on self-preservation skills. You can learn something from all of them. When it comes to self-defence and self-protection, the more strategies you use the better are your chances of success and survival.

One of the most important findings was that when a woman used physical force as a defence technique together with another technique, her chances of escape and survival increased. No woman in our study used physical force alone. In fact, the more additional strategies she used, the greater were her chances. (Bart & O'Brien, p. 34.)

It's important to keep your mind open to all possibilities and to trust yourself if a situation doesn't feel right. The contents of this book will help you to firmly establish and develop feelings of self-love, self-esteem and self-respect. They will help you to enforce your right to control your own body, as well as your right to stop anyone who attempts to prevent you from doing so. This does not mean that you will always be safe, but it will prepare you to deal better, and provide you with the inner resources to deal more wisely and appropriately, with threatening situations.

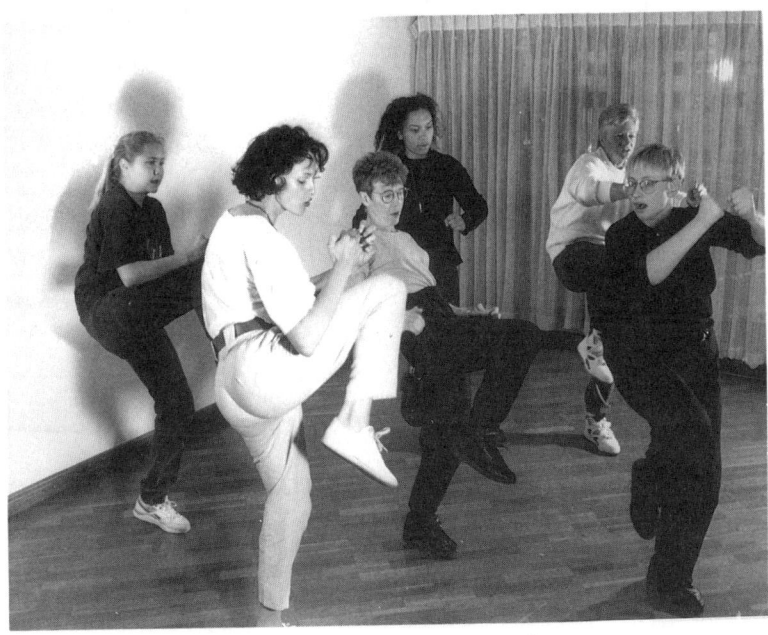

Class learning kneestrike

chapter 2

Bread and butter:
Basic strikes

Striking, is the bread and butter of your defence strategy. Inflicting pain on an attacker is the most effective form of distraction. It's much better to strike the assailant in a direct and pointed way in a vulnerable area than to struggle. So when in doubt, strike and strike hard. Strike suddenly and strike immediately at the vulnerable areas. Remember that striking power can be related more to how rapidly you contract your muscle than to the size of your muscle.

PUNCHING, STRIKING, KICKING
Standard punch
If you contract the muscle very rapidly you're likely to be more effective. By slipping slightly forward as you punch, you can put your body weight behind you and maximise your power. When you punch, get your breath coordinated with your muscular contraction.

First put your hands up and hold them facing out. Fold your fingers over once, twice and then put your thumb over your first two fingers.

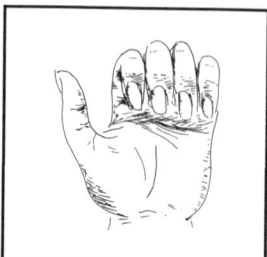 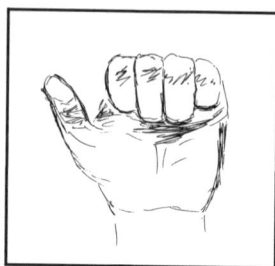 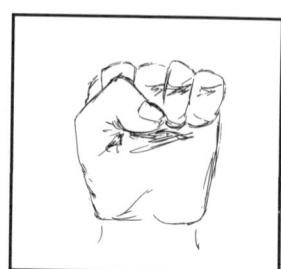

Your hands are up in front of your face, your elbows are facing the ground. What you're going to do is punch slowly towards the centre, in alignment with your own chin, as if you're standing in front of the mirror and hitting yourself on the chin. So you're pushing, hitting and striking with the first joint knuckles towards the chin and then you're pulling your fist back and repeating this with the other fist.

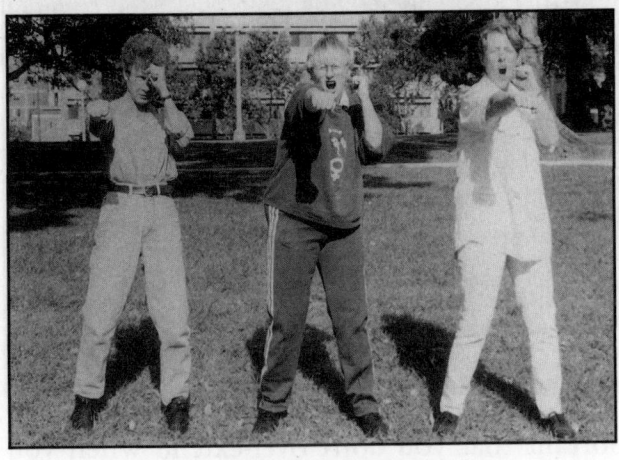

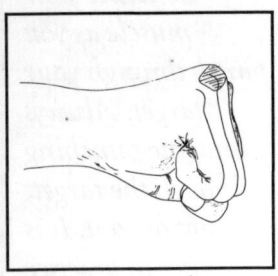

Left: *Yell 'No!' as you strike out. Punch and guard with your other arm*
Right: *Strike primarily with your first two knuckles*

Now put your hands by your sides and breathe out as if you're whispering, contracting your muscles as if there were a bolt of electricity going through your body. So as you contract your muscles you're breathing like this — 'ha' (as if you are breathing garlic into someone's face). So you breathe out and contract and imagine there's a bolt of electricity going through your body. Lift one hand up and place it straight in front of you in alignment with your solar plexus (the centre of the body directly beneath the breast-bone). This is as far as you need to extend.

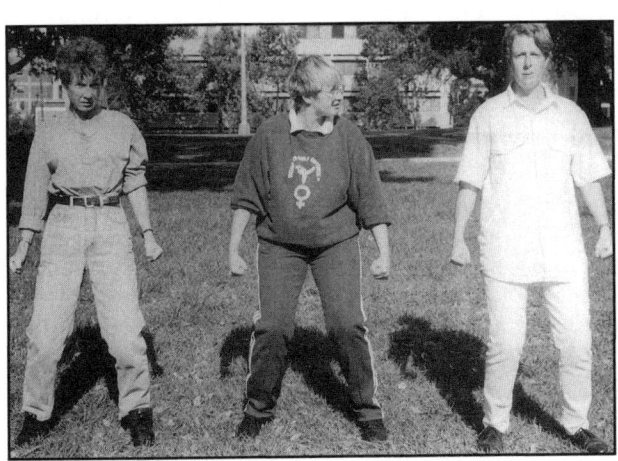

Imagining a bolt of electricity assisting you as you clench your fists to strike

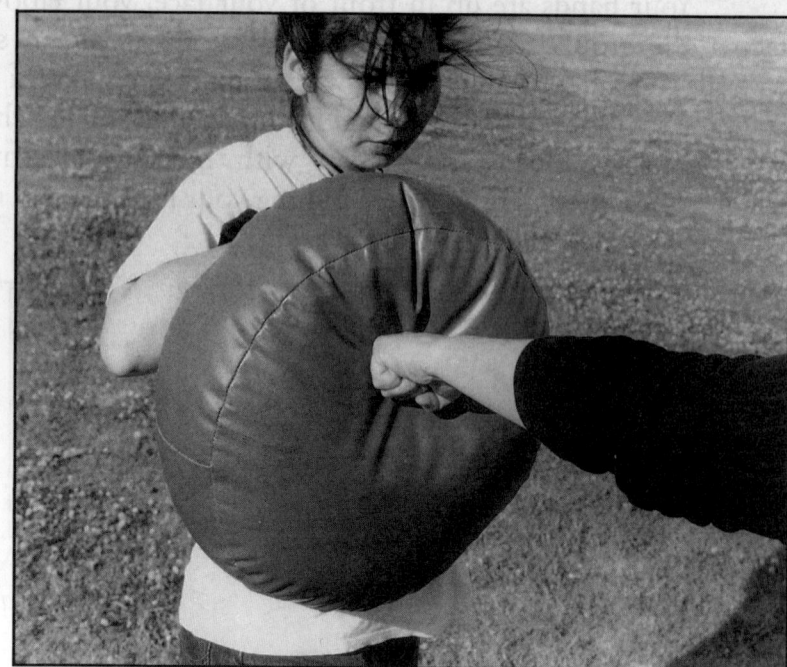

Contract your muscle as you punch through your target. Always imagine punching through the target, not onto it. It is safer to practice with a soft target rather than punching the air

It's very important that you don't over-extend when you punch in the air to the point that you feel your joints cracking or experience pain. When you punch out, you should not feel any of your joints cracking — not your shoulder, not your elbow nor your wrist. If you do experience any pain then be sure to shorten the punch. Instead of punching out 180 degrees, only punch out 170 degrees or whatever you can manage without feeling pain, since you should not feel any discomfort nor any pain after delivering the punch. Your joints should not feel as if they are pulling out of their sockets.

Now pull your hand back. You're going to punch out, contracting the muscle at the end of the punch. Then you're going to pull your arm back as quickly as you push it out, imagining that it's being drawn back by a piece of elastic stretched along the tendon. From there it's a matter of pushing out and pulling your fist back very quickly. That's how you punch: there's the rapid contraction at the end as you breathe out, there's the sense of electricity that helps to bring the punching fist back as quickly as it goes out, ensuring that it will travel back along the same path that it travelled out on. Of course, in a real-life situation the circumstances will vary greatly and so will the way that you punch, but this initial description of how to punch provides a starting point from which to ground yourself.

Breath, noise and movement

Imagine a magic button located two inches below your navel. Some people call this your chi or ki centre. You might call it your 'no' button. Push this sharply and yell 'No' in a deep, well-projected baritone voice. ('No' is an easier sound to make than a more traditional martial arts yell.) This sound will ignite your warrior spirit and centre you for the task ahead. Now you can focus your energies whilst seeming out of control to an observer. Then make your facial expression match your inner-centredness with a don't-mess-with-me-unless-you-want-trouble look.

Don't let your 'No' get high-pitched and stuck in the throat. It should remain baritone and come from deep within you. If you want to use a different word to 'No', feel free to do so. As you start to emit your 'kia' (this is the Japanese name for the sound you are making), you first imagine it going out one foot in front of you. The next time it goes three feet, then across the room, across the street, around the world, then throughout the universe. Let your 'aura' (the invisible force field that protects you) expand with the sound. Feel that you are occupying an ever-increasing amount of space (see the exercises below); feel a sense of your body loosening and expanding.

Now we want to co-ordinate all these elements and make them work together. As you punch, I want you to 'kia', breathe, expand your aura and project your facial expression so that you are working as a total physical, emotional and spiritual unit, co-ordinating your power with absolute commitment. You can then use this process to accompany all of your strikes once you have a basic idea as to how they are coordinated on a purely physical level.

Knee to the groin strike

If somebody grabs you, you can immediately grab them and come in, pushing in with the top of the knee, not the knee itself, but the top part of the knee. Come in, grab the person and then knee their groin, solar plexus or face (see photograph on p. 37).

The attacker's neck or arms can be held to keep balance and generate power forward. It's more the top of the knee that you use in this strike. Striking once with the knee may not be enough to achieve your purpose, so after the initial kick, drop the ball of your foot to the ground, push off the ground in a bouncing motion. First strike the groin, then return to the ground, then bounce up to hit the solar plexus, return to the ground, then up to the face. I

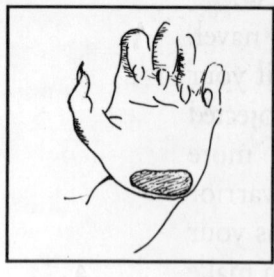

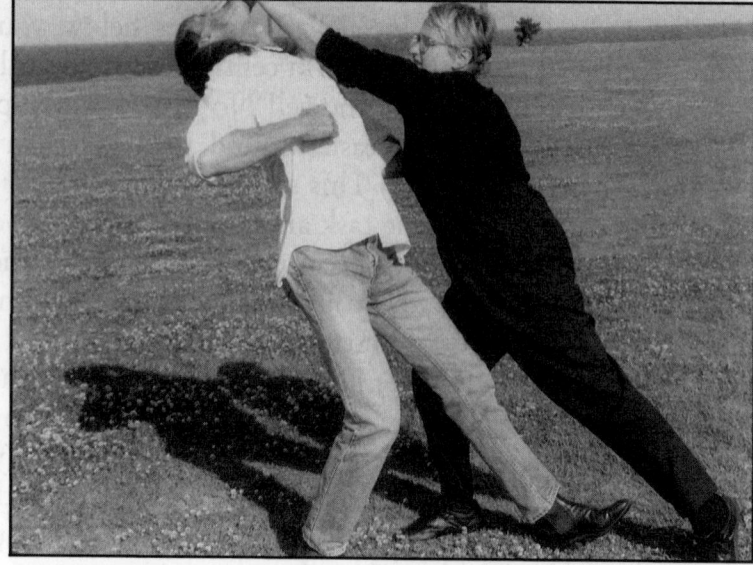

Heel of palm strike. Keep a wide stance and move with the attacker's force

call this 'bouncy knees'. The heel is kept as close to the buttocks as possible, giving the knee a sharp point with which to strike.

Heel of palm strike
Come in towards the attacker with your fingers facing slightly backward, that is, towards the ceiling, keeping them slightly backward. You're hitting with the heel of the palm either coming straight up under the chin or straight up under the nose. As you strike your fingers curve in a concave motion and strike like a cat into the eyes before pulling back.

Elbow strike
Think of using a turning-the-tap-on, turning-the-tap-off motion. First of all turn your feet in a T-stance, so that one foot is facing toe-in toward the other one, like a T, but at least a shoulder-width apart.

The foot facing in rests on the ball of the foot with its heel raised off the ground. Next you reverse it, so that the foot with the heel off the ground is now flat, and the other foot has its heel off the ground, always keeping the T-formation. Think of an Elvis Presley movement: one foot up, one foot down, one foot up, one foot down. When the right heel is up, raise the right elbow and turn your body around, turning your right foot in a T-motion towards the left foot. So the elbow will come across your centre-line, and then as it recrosses the line it will drop in by your chest.

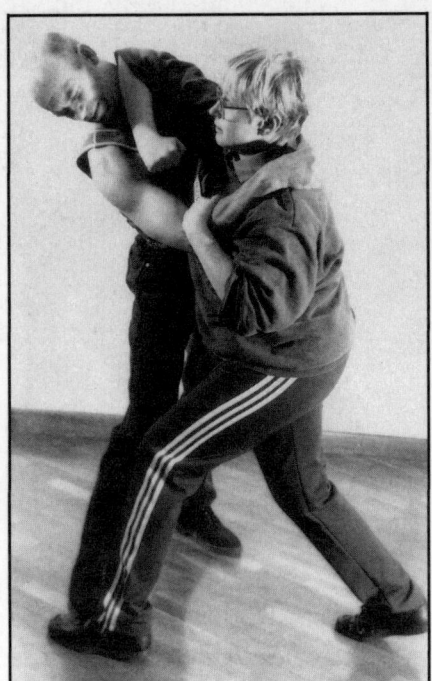 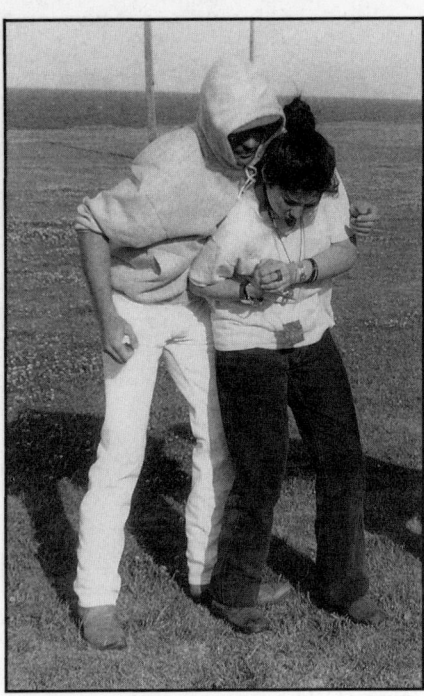

Left: *As you 'turn the tap on' you can use this movement to strike, break a hold, or distract. Turn your feet in a T-stance so your foot faces the direction you are striking in. Rotating the feet allows you to put your entire body into the technique.* Right: *Elbow strike to the rear. Use one hand to hold the other for added strength*

Bear in mind that this strike is similar to a turning-the-tap-on, turning-the-tap-off motion, but the body is part of the tap. In this tap movement, your feet are the faucet and your arms are the tap. You make your feet and arms coordinate with one another. So you are not just using arm-strength, but the power of your whole body working as a unit in one direction.

This movement has a variety of applications. It can be used as a strike by bringing the elbow into the jaw, solar plexus, or throat. It may be used as a hold-breaker by directing the elbows diagonally, or if for some reason the person is too strong, or is bracing you against a wall and you find it difficult to break the hold in this way, it may be used to distract by getting them to concentrate on your upper body while you then kick them very hard in the groin (several times if necessary). Remember if one thing isn't working you just try something else. It's not the technique that works, it's you working the technique that works!

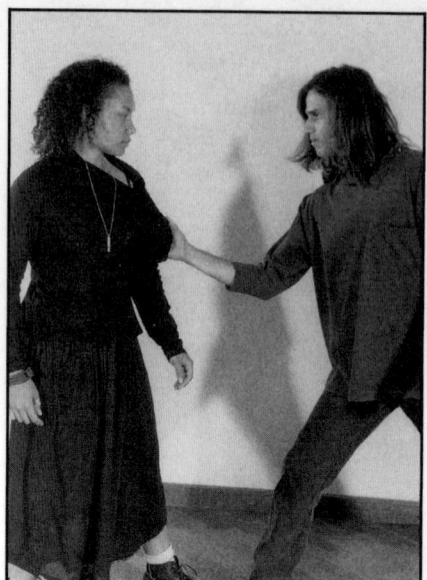 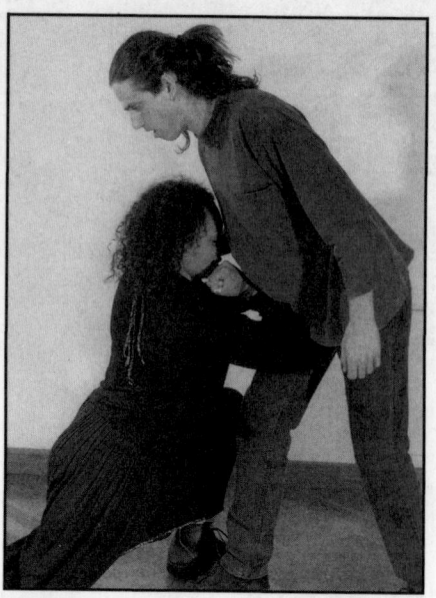

Left: *Being grabbed — you have several options*. Right: *If pulled to the ground, one option is to strike the groin with the elbow to the midline (groin). The same technique can be used if standing to strike the solar plexus or face*

Elbow strike to the rear

This is useful if someone has grabbed you from behind. First, displace your hip, so that you're off the centre-line and you're striking in with the elbow straight back into the solar plexus, groin or whatever you can hit at the centre-line of the person behind you. Move the hip out of the way and strike with the elbow straight behind you.

To reinforce this element you can close the fist of the striking hand, grasping it with the other hand to drive it backwards and reinforce the motion backwards.

A student of mine broke the ribs of another student practising this, from which you can conclude: 1) you must use control when practising with a training partner; and 2) this works! P.S. If they have a beer-gut aim lower.

Elbow to midline strike

Step forward with your elbow moving up in a perpendicular motion, coming straight up in the air. Come in straight at the solar plexus, the jaw, the groin, basically at anything you can hit, but make sure you don't hit yourself on the way up. The little finger brushes against the ear as it comes up in a perpendicular motion and as you step forward. So as you step forward and as your body weight lands, so does the technique, allowing you to put all your body weight behind it. Remember that stepping forward as you land a strike is a very direct way of magnifying your power. Whether you are using an elbow, knee, fist, club, stapler or whatever, put your entire body weight behind it.

One of my senior students, who is 69 years old, used her body to great effect. She was walking down a busy street in the middle of the day when she became aware that she was being followed. (Obviously her early warning signs had been heightened by having completed less than half of a twelve-week course.) Eventually she turned around and confronted him, asking, 'What do you want?' He replied, 'Money'. She replied, 'I haven't got any money, and I wouldn't give it to you even if I did'. He then proceeded to put his hands in his pockets. At that point my student was fearful that he was about to pull out a weapon. So she raised her fist, dropped her body weight forward and punched him right in the jaw, knocking him to the ground. She then said, 'And if you get up I'll give you another one!' When she told me this story, I felt euphoric. At that time there was a psychopath who had already murdered two older women (and went on to kill more) in the suburbs, and here was an elderly woman standing up for herself.

Let's consider all of the weapons that my student used beyond just the punch. Because she was aware of being followed, she was not taken by surprise. Her early warning detector generated an intuitive response: she turned around and confronted her would-be assailant directly. Note that this is not always the appropriate action, so unfortunately we can make no clear rules about this. She anticipated his next move and so caught him unaware when his hands were in his pockets, hit him on a sensitive point (the jaw) with 100 per cent commitment, resolute intention, and with all her body weight behind what she was doing. As you can see, she used more than just one strategy.

Elbow to the side strike
Somebody is running at you. Lift your elbow up and strike into the side, the jaw or whatever you can. Remember to breathe out, pretending there's a bolt of electricity going through your body, sharply contracting your muscle as though penetrating and driving through your target.

One of my students completed a 12-week course with me some years ago. She then studied Tae Kwon Do for a year or so.

One night she found herself in the middle of a pub brawl with a large man running toward her, a mean look in his eye. She promptly lifted her elbow in the above-mentioned way, hit the man in the face and knocked him out. As she told me this victorious tale she expressed her own surprise at using something that she had learned over twelve months before rather than anything she had recently learnt. The point here is that in most situations your attacker will be too close for you to use a long-range technique, so it's very important to learn very simple techniques that work at short-range.

If someone has both of their hands on you and is pulling you by one of your arms, maybe into a car or alley, a good strategy

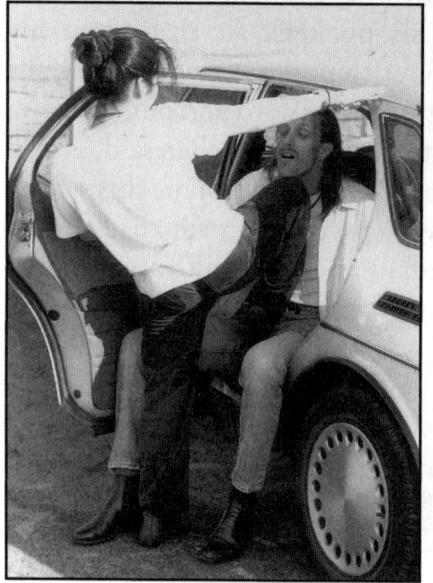 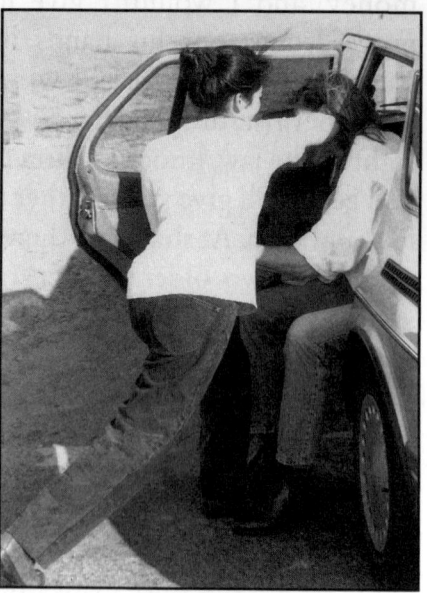

Left: If someone is dragging you into a car, move forward, get your stability and strike them in a vulnerable spot. Get your balance by moving with their force and widening your stance — then run!
Right: An elbow strike to the jaw can be effective; for most women this will have more impact than a simple punch

is to resist a little in the opposite direction, then when the attacker is pulling you good and hard, use the momentum this gives you to launch a fist, elbow, knee, finger, heel of palm into an exposed vulnerable area. That is, use the other person's power, plus your own against the attacker. (Remember to stabilise yourself. Keep your feet wide apart and bend your knees so as to maintain your balance. This applies to most attacks where someone is trying to throw you off balance. Also remember that you can mix-and-match vulnerable areas with the 'weapons' you have on your body and, if you can find an external weapon eg. pen, stapler, lamp, dirt, all the better.)

Snap kick

As your leg comes up, lift your knee and flick with the flat of the top of your foot. The knee should come up the centre of your body to at least navel-height, in alignment with your navel. Remember that the spot your knee points at is the spot you will kick, so your knee must point like the sight on a gun. If the knee is crooked, then you will deliver a crooked hit at your target.

The top of the foot is flat, toes pointing down. Your Achilles' tendon is scrunched up at the back. Do not kick with your toes. Aim at the scrotum, not the penis, kicking with a snapping motion. It's not a power kick so much as an accuracy kick because it won't hurt anything if you don't actually connect with the groin area. (My editor asked, 'What if the attacker is a woman?' My answer is that it still hurts a lot – a hard kick can fracture the pubic bone.)

This kick is appropriate if someone has their legs apart, since it must hit in an upward motion into the testicles, but this

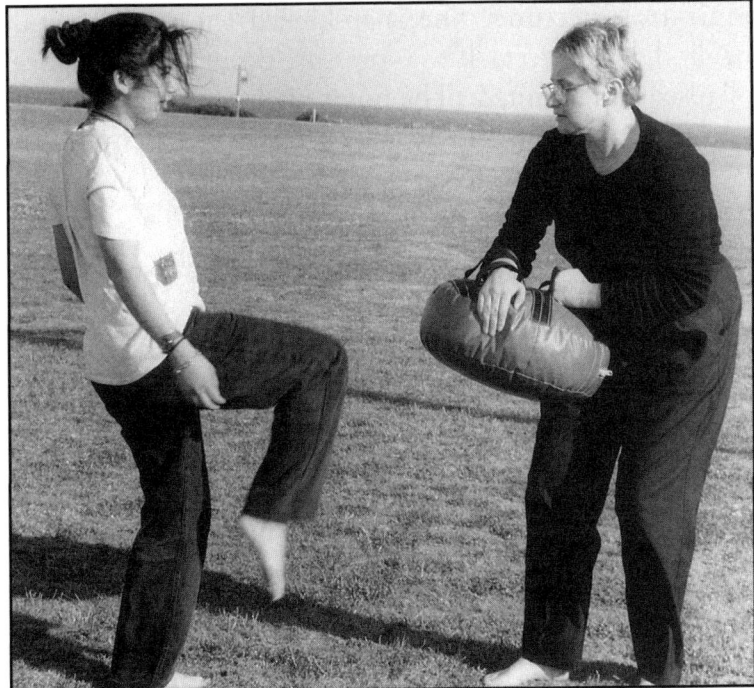

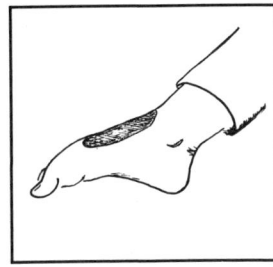

Snap kick – strike with the flat of the top of the foot. Lift your knee up in line with the target. Use it like the sight of a gun; point your knee where you want your kick to go

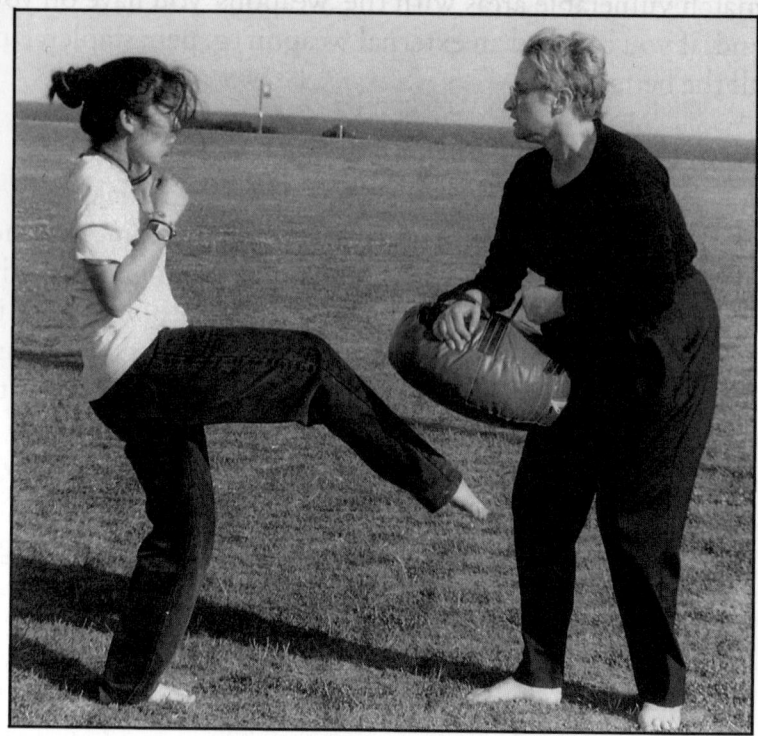

The snap kick is done as a flicking motion up between the legs. Snap quickly back so your leg cannot be grabbed

kick is useless if the attacker's legs are together. (For attackers who stand with their legs together, see the next kick.)

In one incident a university student was grabbed as she was walking home from lectures. She snap-kicked the testicles and pubic bone and, I suspect, hit a pressure-point, because her attacker collapsed and vomited. (The point of all of these stories, is always to assess your options and not rely on only one technique.)

Front kick

Lift the knee up and, with your toes back, deliver the kick with the ball of the foot. Push your hips forward as you thrust your leg. The energy of this kick is horizontal. You're pushing straight in with the hips, coming in with the ball of the foot to the groin or on the hip. If it lands higher on the body it can be quite effective in pushing the person back. This kick can be used with either a pushing energy or a hitting energy and will have an effect wherever it lands on the body. If you are in a position where you can't use close-range techniques, a front kick may be particularly useful.

Another of my students, a woman of about thirty years, used a front kick to great effect after having only one lesson. In the

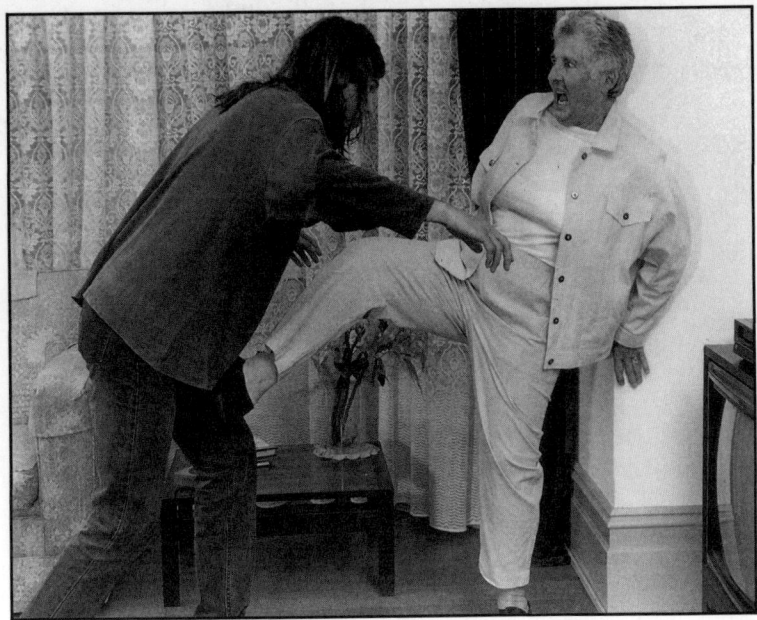
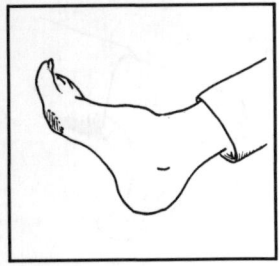

Front kick to the attacker's groin. Keep the toes back and kick with the ball of the foot. If possible, balance yourself by holding onto a wall or fixed object to give you more stability

middle of a custody battle her ex-husband attempted to forcibly take the kids. He had put them in the car. Enraged, she kicked a big dent in the car with a front kick, opened the car door, grabbed the kids out of the car, and, as her six-foot ex was coming forward, front-kicked him in the mid-section catapulting him several feet backward against a fence. There he stayed with a stunned mullet expression on his face, not able to comprehend how his five-foot ex-wife had managed to kick him backward with such force whilst she was clutching two small children! She hadn't hit him in a vital area, but the kick still had the desired effect.

Side kick (angling downward)
From the side, bring your heel to your buttocks. Your toes are facing in towards you as you thrust down diagonally on to the kneecap or, preferably, to the side of the knee. This kick can also be dealt with the blade of the foot and can be aimed anywhere on the body, however the knee joint is the most accessible target. When you are practising this kick, aiming it at your partner's cushion or punching bag held at knee-height (see Exercise 2 below), be careful! The bag holder should keep their knees bent and the bag in front of them. This is an effective kick; the stopping effect can cause considerable pain, even through a hand-held punching bag.

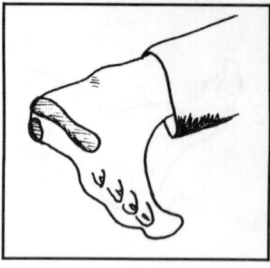
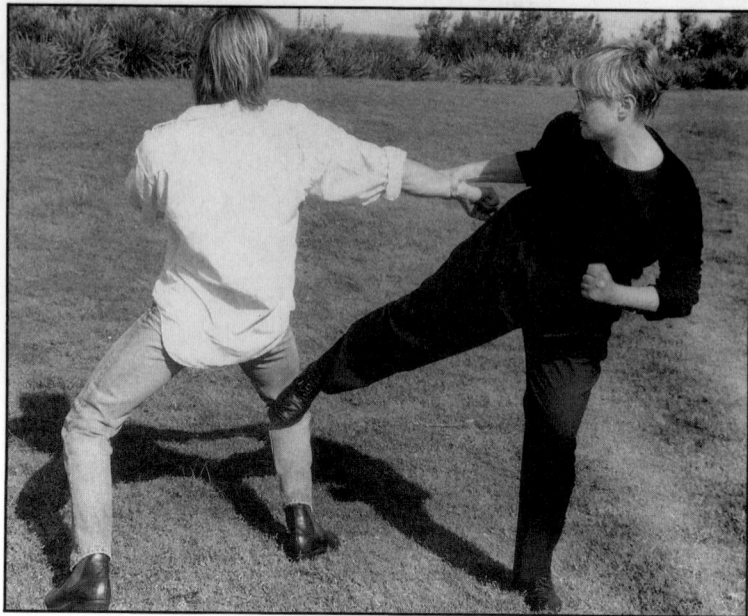

Stomp through behind the attacker's knee with your heel or side of foot

Front heel kick

Come in, lifting the knee up at the front and strike with the heel in a straight-line motion, straight in under the kneecap, preferably to the side of the knee or where the knee is slightly bent. If you're wearing high heels, aim the kick at the groin or just about anywhere. You can use this kick just to get space for yourself and get someone away from you.

With this kick it is better to hit the knee when the knee is straight and not locked in a bent position. This is because the knee is very strong when slightly bent and, unless you hit it on an angle, that is, on the side or the back of the knee, all you may end up hurting is your foot. So if someone stands facing you slightly pigeon-toed, then they are in a perfect position to be hit in the inner knee, but if their knees are facing you and if they are bent, you would be better off to kick them hard at the bottom of the shin, particularly if you are wearing hard-soled shoes.

I used this kick when I was in London researching a series of articles on women in the martial arts worldwide. I was wandering with Huggy Bear (the name I gave my koala backpack and security blanket) when an obnoxious drunk started harassing me at a coffee shop, much as he had been bothering everyone in his path. I suppose he thought me a likely target, being short and blonde and feeling a bit forlorn that day with a koala on my back — little did

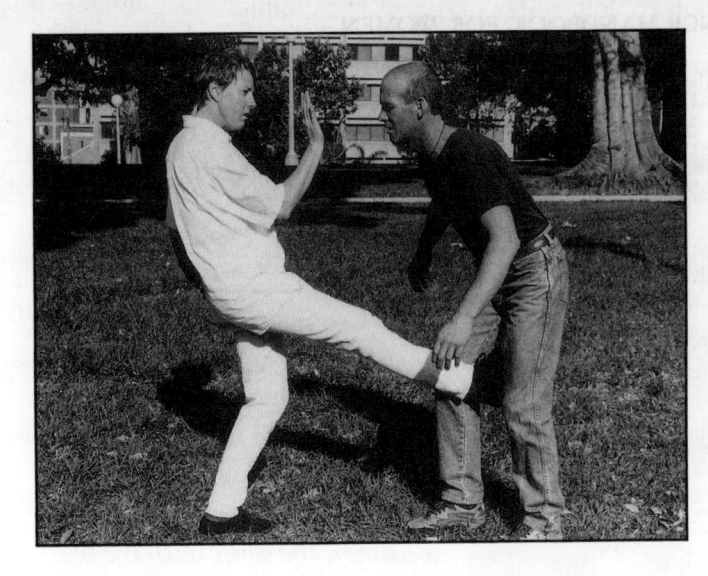

Front heel kick to the inner knee to inflict damage or kick slowly your harasser's bent knee. Reinforce this with hand movements and yell 'No!' to stop low level harassment

he know! As he came toward me I used a front heel kick with a slow muscular contraction, so as to stop him entering my space. I looked him right in the eye and said in my most powerful voice, 'Leave me alone'. He was taken aback by my foot coming out. I think he thought he had run into a chair. He continued to harass me, but from the safe distance of one leg-length away, even after I put my foot down.

Back kick

This is very useful when somebody is behind you. With your knees together, lift one knee up and kick backward with the heel. Your toes are pointing backward, either onto the other person's knee or towards their groin. Sometimes, if you are close, you can actually just flick the kick up: lift the heel straight up, kick backward and pretend you are a kicking horse. With the knees together, kick backward with one leg in a thrusting motion.

The back kick is best practised with your bottom facing your target, looking over your shoulder, but without moving the rest of your body, and then kicking sharply backwards. Experimenting with different distances can help you understand the distance/power relationship.

One schoolgirl I was teaching was attacked on her way to school by three teenagers. A boy grabbed her from behind and she back-kicked him in the groin, causing him to collapse on the ground. She was punched severely in the face by a girl at the front before they fled. The lesson to be learned here is to deal first with the person who is about to hit you — this is usually the person at your front.

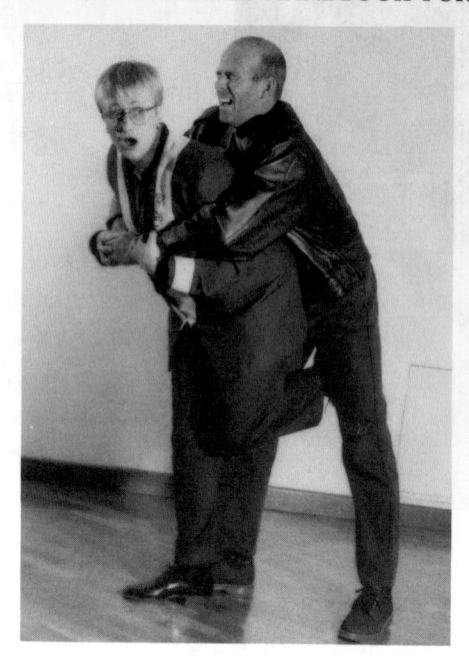

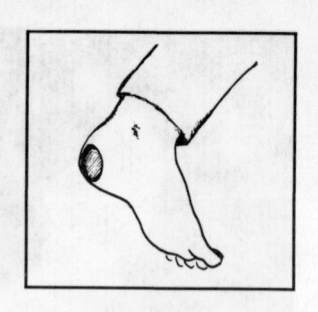

Back kicks will usually be applied as a flick up between the legs with the knee. Alternatively, you could scrape down the shins with the heel and stomp on the attacker's foot

Head-butt

This is not one I would put high on the priority list, but it's definitely an option. If you head-butt, use the back of your head or the top of your forehead at the front (see p. 40). It's more practical to head-butt someone who is taller than you are, so the top of your head moves into their nose and chin. The risk is that this may make you feel a bit concussed, depending on how hard your head is, so I don't recommend it as a primary line of defence.

A well-known self-defence instructor in Washington, DC, Carole Middleton, who has studied karate for over twenty-five years, was accosted by a man in her apartment. He pinned her arms to the wall, so she couldn't use her arms, and he was too close for her to be able to use her feet or knees. She had watched her instructor break ice with his head, so, thinking that she had nothing to lose, she head-butted him on the nose and chin. Blood gushed from the man's face as he collapsed unconscious. She didn't feel a thing.

Remember that striking is useful as a means of distracting your attacker. The more practice you get the more confident you will feel.

MULTIPLE ATTACK

The incidence of multiple attack on women is much less than the incidence of attack from a single assailant. It was found in a survey conducted in the USA that only fourteen per cent of women attacked were attacked by two or more assailants at the one time.

BREAD AND BUTTER: BASIC STRIKES   37

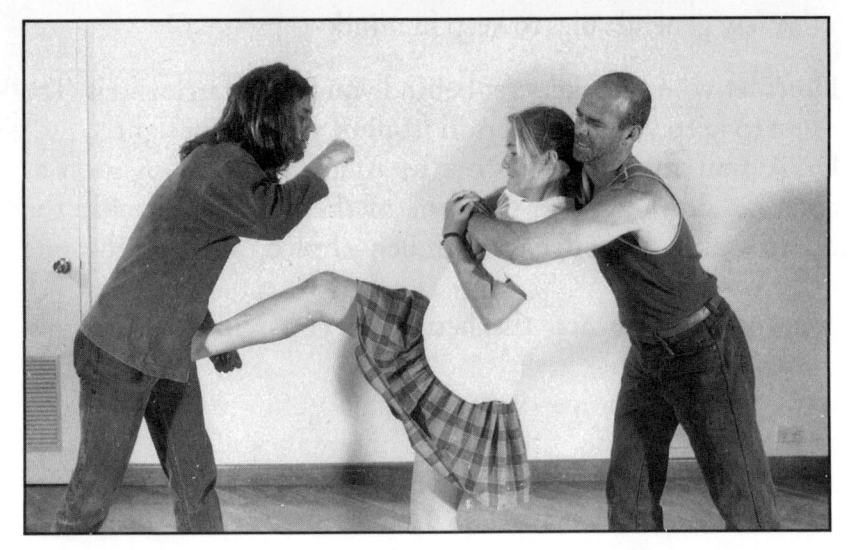

Take out the one most likely to hit you. Hands are held, but she can still kick to the groin. Scream and make as much noise as possible

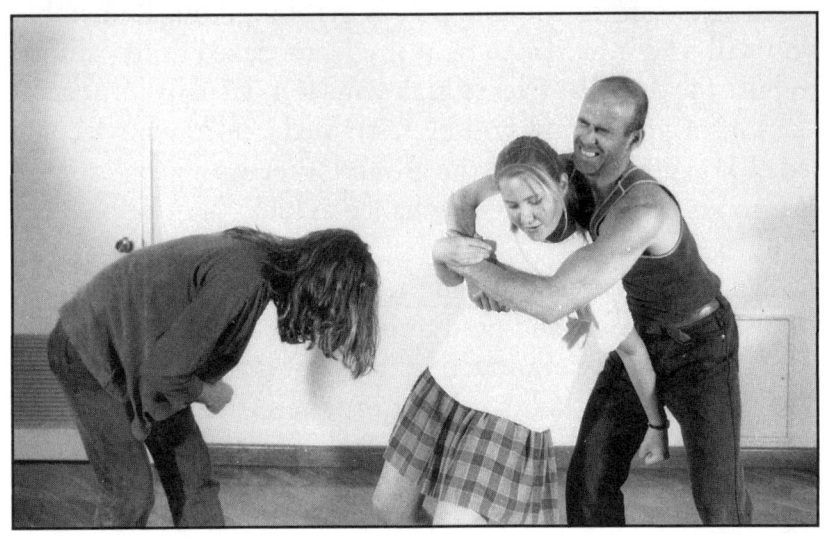

Follow through with a rear strike to the groin

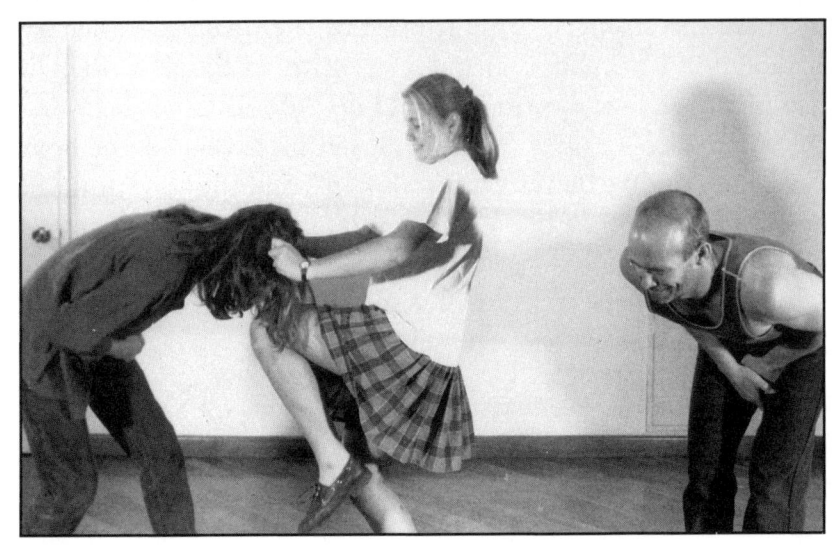

Back again for a knee to the face — best done three times to reach his pain threshold

A few general rules to keep in mind:

1. Don't let your attackers get behind you if you can avoid it. Try your best to keep your attackers in front of you and in sight.
2. Don't wait for the aggressors to attack you. Try as soon as possible, i.e. don't wait, to take one of them out, preferably the leader. However, if you haven't much choice, aim for the one closest to you.
3. The quicker you act, the better off you will be. Action is quicker than reaction.
4. If you have a choice or can arrange it, try to handle your attackers one at a time. Often only one man will grab you first because they don't expect strong resistance.
5. Always try to hurt the one that looks like they might hit you first, then take care of the one that is grabbing you. Remember that you will find it harder to fight if you are dazed or in pain. Be sure to hurt the one that tries to grab your feet. Usually your arms and the top of your body will be restrained before your feet are grasped or you are brought to the ground. Feet are a gang's second priority, so you will usually get a chance to kick them before they grab your legs.
6. Make noise, resist, persist and the more of them there are, the more noise you'll want and need to make. Try to get someone to intervene. If you see a gang attack someone, it is a good ploy to call out 'The police are on their way'. For instance, there was a worker in a youth detention centre who was attacked by four youths at the centre late one afternoon. They wrestled her to the ground with the intention of raping her. One held each limb. She said she didn't know where the strength came from, but she lifted back her leg (she had on heavy army boots) and let go with an almighty kick to the face of the guy attempting to hold down one of her legs. She felt his face crumple under the force of her foot. One of the boys panicked and said 'We better get out of here', and they all took off. Group attackers are not brave and can be easy to disperse if you disrupt their plan.
7. A lot of multiple attacks involve someone luring you to a spot where a group is waiting for you — be careful!

Here are some exercises to help you focus on the concepts in this chapter. I would advise that you use someone who respects your commitment and does not ridicule your efforts as you work through these exercises.

Exercise 1

With a partner, match all the strikes in this chapter with all the vulnerable areas in the photograph. Notice what effect the size you are has upon distancing and position in these techniques. This exercise starts to lock into your memory exactly where the vital striking points are. Do the strikes slowly and analyse their potential effect. Don't start punching and kicking each other; this exercise is to work on your mind. You are storing the strikes there, ready to be drawn upon whenever your personal safety is jeopardised.

Exercise 2

Get a pillow or cushion or, if your budget permits, you may want to invest in a hand-held punching bag. Before beginning you can record this short centering exercise on tape and then play it to yourself:

- Close your eyes. Imagine someone is attacking you in the way in which you can use a punch (or other technique). Breathe deeply. Imagine you are inhaling courage, exhaling fear, inhaling strength, exhaling weakness, inhaling self-love, exhaling self-hate, inhaling faith in your ability, exhaling doubt, inhaling power, exhaling powerlessness, inhaling hope, exhaling hopelessness.
- Then imagine a clear white light coming from the sky or ceiling, coming down through the top of your head – an incredible energy source permeating your whole body, igniting your 'No' button and, from this centralised spot, sending a strong powerful, irradiating energy through all the limbs of your body.
- Open your eyes. Now slowly punch into the bag to make sure you are doing it correctly. Then imagine that the light is helping your fist go right through the bag.
- For the person holding it, make sure you are standing side-on, with your feet wide apart, bracing the cushion on your hip and moving your head right out of the way of the cushion.
- A free-standing light punching bag which can be hung from the ceiling is an excellent practise tool, if you have somewhere to put it. As you punch, incorporate your kia noise, rapid muscular contraction, breathing, facial expression, light, energy and forward-intention through the bag. Remember to rapidly withdraw your fist after you have penetrated your target.

Head-butt or strike with the top of your forehead against his chin or nose. If you are much shorter, you can come up under his chin and push upwards

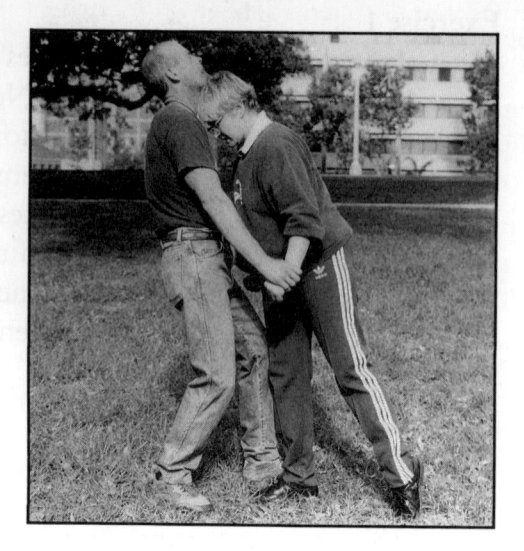

- Remember that, if you are going to bother hitting someone, make it count! Now do the same with the kicks and punches, but make sure that you hit the bag, not the person holding the bag, because you are a lot more powerful than you think you are!
- Do each technique slowly, first to make sure you are aware of exactly where you are hitting, and that the person holding the bag has placed it in the correct spot.

Exercise 3
Once you have mastered these simple techniques, combine them so that they land on different levels of the body, going from high to low, and from low to high, alternating right and left, using both your hands and feet.

For instance, left heel palm strike to the face, right perpendicular elbow strike to the mid-section, left knee to the groin, or right leg back-kick to groin, left elbow moving backward to solar plexus, right elbow swinging around to head.

Again I remind you to do these exercises slowly at first, and only strike at a pace that allows the person holding the cushion to move it into a protective position in time.

You can also experiment with distancing.

Exercise 4
- This is easier to do if there are several of you. Have two people hold your arms and another person hold a target (cushion or punching bag) while you kick multi-directionally aiming for

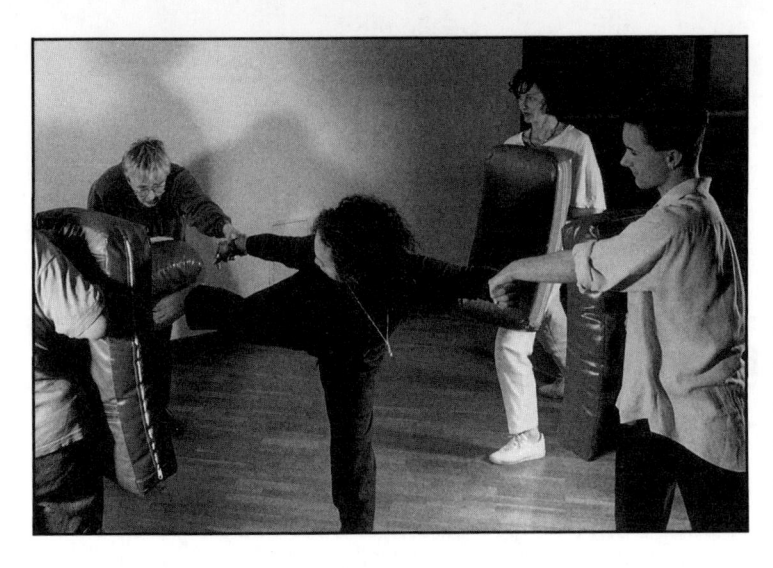

Practice kicking multi-directionally onto soft targets. This exercise can be done with large cushions at home or in a class

the target. I emphasise kicks here because your arms will be the first part of the body to be restrained, leaving only your legs to do the work. Try this exercise also without being held down.
- Stand in the middle of a circle of people and assess where you would hit them, striking them in slow motion, focusing on the target.
- If you are alone you can still practise kicking backwards, to the front, to the side and from the ground. Practise changing position. Yell 'No' as you do this. Practise making a ruckus, see how long you can keep this up without getting tired. (If your neighbours come in to see what's going on, you know you have succeeded.)
- Practise being a bowling ball on the ground. Grab people's legs, keep moving and bowl them over, give them a kick or two if they come in range. Still don't let them get near your head.

SUMMARY
- Strike vulnerable areas of the body – e.g. eyes, throat, groin.
- Yell 'No' as you strike.
- Get your balance.
- Use your body weight to reinforce the strike.
- Strike as often as it takes (persistence momentum).

chapter 3

Attacks from the front

From the front of her house Linda saw a man sitting with his legs protruding from the open passenger door of a dirty white Holden car parked along the street. 'He was dragging into the car a dark-haired woman who was screaming,' Linda said. 'He had hold of her by the arm and shoulder and I could see she was trying to get away. She was trying to struggle free.'
(Julia Sheppard, *Someone Else's Daughter: The Life and Death of Anita Cobby*, Ironbark Press, Sydney, 1991.)

Attacks can come from any direction. It's virtually impossible to predict exactly how or from what direction one might be attacked or what strikes might serve you best at the time. However, you are more likely to be attacked from behind (see next chapter) and there are some commonly known attack positions — bearhugs, choke holds and mugger's holds. Most attack situations are unclear, consisting of untidy grappling energy which may involve several different grabs in a matter of seconds. Thus experimentation in the form of the exercises at the end of this chapter is vital to achieving a clear understanding of what you could encounter and how you might react to and deal with it.

BALANCE may be achieved by widening your stance and bending your knees to lower your centre of gravity. If you are being forced in a certain direction, you may have to take several large steps in that direction in order to accommodate a large force coming at you (see Exercise 1 at the end of the chapter).

We must keep our strategies, outlined in Chapter 1, in the forefront of our minds when we are grappling with a larger, stronger attacker. Remember you cannot deal with a stronger opponent on his terms, because if you try to you will come out only second best. Recall that your own range of strategies include screaming, spitting, striking, and reasoning. Always be determined and play as dirty as you have to, targeting particularly the eyes, throat and groin with your strikes.

Being choked from the front

1. The first thing you must do is pull your chin firmly down and in toward your throat the moment you feel pressure of any kind on your neck.
2. Step backward in a wide stance and sink low if you're being pushed backward.
3. Strike a vulnerable exposed area to loosen your attacker up a bit. (See diagram in Chapter 2.)
4. Bring your arms up on top of the attacker's. Pivot on one foot in toward the other, as you swivel the adjacent elbow downwards diagonally in a turn-the-tap-on, turn-the-tap-off motion (see Chapter 2). Move your body as if you are attempting to turn right around.

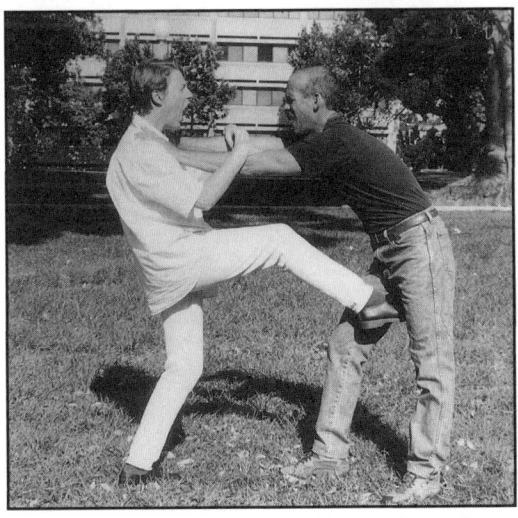

Put you chin down, yell, and strike a vulnerable area

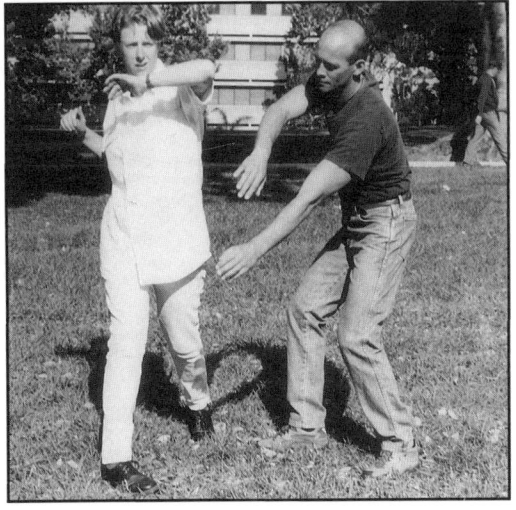

Twist your feet with your elbows in a turning the tap motion to strike, hold, break or distract

The striking distraction is particularly important if an attacker has you pinned against a wall, because the wall supports and effectively increases the strength of the attacker's grip. An instructor from our academy researched this the hard way when a man, whom she was attempting to remove from a nightclub where she worked, pinned her to the wall by the throat. She had to snap kick him three times hard in the groin before he let her go.

Remember that all of these actions work best when reinforced with noise and emotional commitment. Being grabbed by the throat is a sure way of evoking fear, especially when this action is accompanied by threatening statements such as, 'Keep quiet or I'll kill you', specifically designed to play on the victim's fear of death – easily done in these circumstances. Recreating as much as possible these threatening situations and rehearsing or practising a response can help to put aside some of the emotional fear associated with this sort of attack (See Exercise 1).

Being grabbed by one arm

In this instance your attacker has severely underestimated your capacity to fight back, is engaging you in low-level harassment, and is about to strike you or has a weapon.

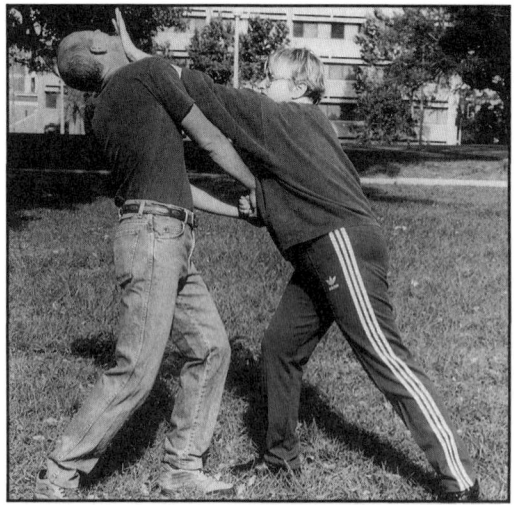

He's got your hand, but your other hand is free – here a heel of palm strike is employed

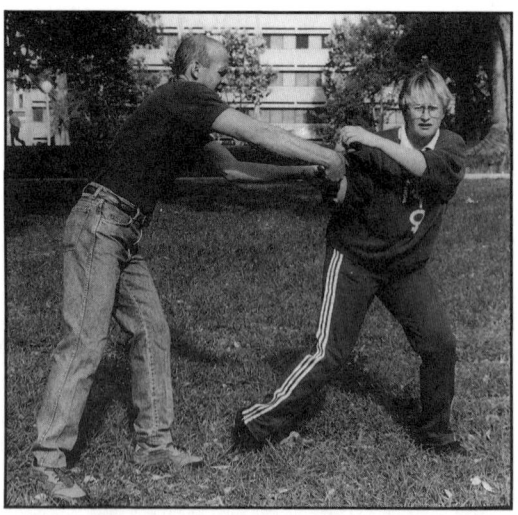

If it is just low-level harassment you may only want to pull your arm away. Make your feet move in the direction you want to go

Your strategy:

1. Scream, strike vulnerable area.
2. Reach over the top of the attacker's hand and grab your other hand, clench your two hands together in a fist position, pulling your fists in a turn-the-tap-on, turn-the-tap-off motion; always cross over the top of the attacker's arm and throw your full body weight behind the turn; this technique will work for any single-arm grab.

Being grabbed by the leg

As soon as someone goes to grab your leg or knee, knee them in the head, because they usually have to bend down to reach your lower limbs.

Frontal bear hug

If someone is squeezing you hard with your arms pinned by your sides:

1. Reach in, grab the scrotum and squeeze as hard as possible. You can get a feel for this strategy by practising at home with two squash balls. Squeeze vigorously, and keep your house-mates guessing what you're up to! Other options are head-butting and foot-stomping.
2. Put two hands on his hips and push yourself backwards.
3. Knee as hard as possible in the groin – to knee someone in the groin there needs to be a little distance between you and your attacker. If someone holds you out at a distance, you must strike them with a longer-range technique – front kick or side kick.

In a front-on attack you have more chance to see your attacker coming. It may be a situation which you have anticipated through a build-up of circumstances. I was attacked on a midnight jog around an inner-city park. I saw a young man jogging toward me. I wasn't wearing my glasses and didn't recognise him but assumed that he must know me. He ran up and grabbed both of my wrists front-on in a wide stance and said authoritatively, 'Keep quiet'. I immediately started to struggle, emitting those primal noises that are totally involuntary, and somehow ended up on my knees, hitting frantically backwards in the air. At this point my attacker made a hasty exit. This occurred shortly after I had started attending self-defence classes and I certainly wasn't experienced enough to use any clear or precise techniques, but the fact that I had resisted nosily and vigorously was enough to have my assailant making tracks.

You will notice a common theme running through the success and effectiveness of all of these techniques. Even if you do them only vaguely right, so long as you KEEP striking, kicking, screaming, and swinging your limbs dynamically, the overall effect is likely to prove a powerful deterrent. Remember it's not WHAT you do but HOW you do it.

Being grabbed with two hands on your two hands

This usually gives you a clear line of attack with the knee to the groin because most attackers open their legs wide to stabilise themselves (the ones I train with do anyway).

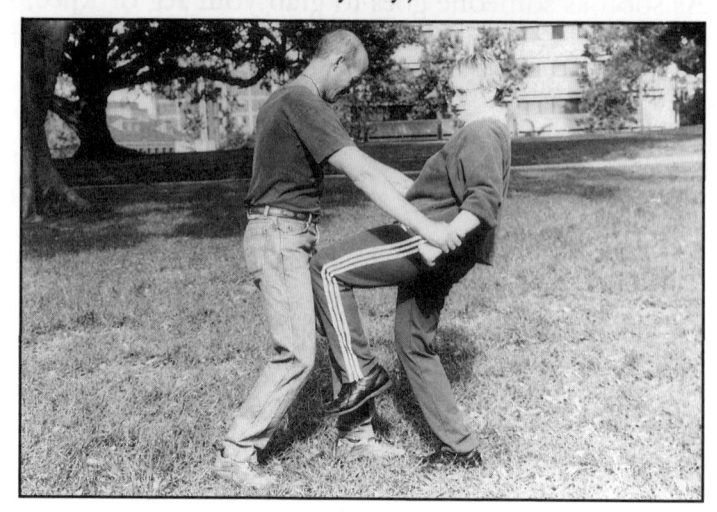

1. Stabilise your own stance
2. Strike to the groin

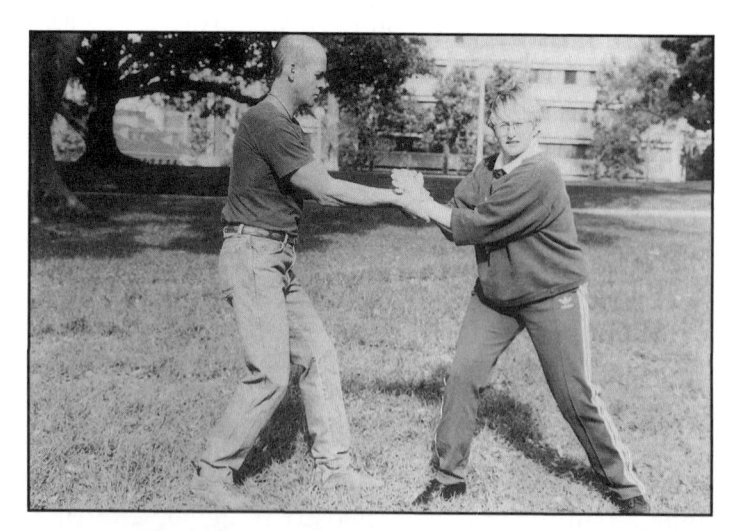

3. Extend your elbows horizontally
4. Grasp hands together and turn your body away from the attacker

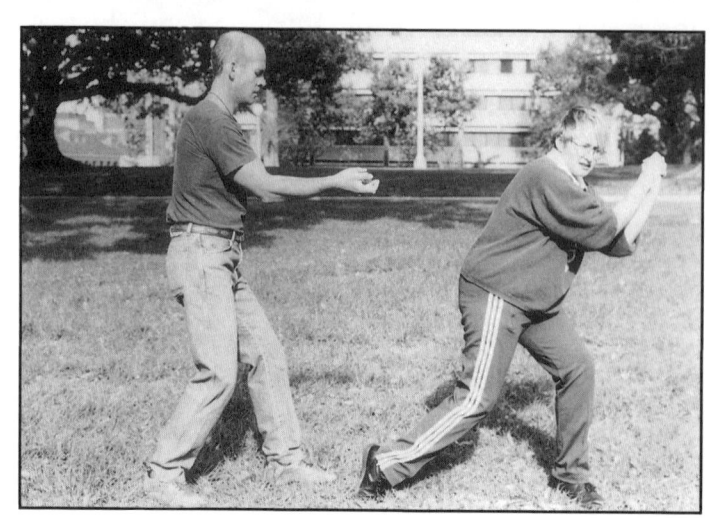

5. Turn your body and arms in a turn-the-tap-on motion. Turn your feet in the direction you want to go; in this instance, away from the attacker

Hair pulling

This is something commonly done to women and can be very painful.

1. As soon as your hair is grabbed, don't pull away but push down on the attacker's hands with both of yours.
2. Establish your balance (if standing) in the direction you are being pulled.
3. Cover your face with your arms in case he is going to hit you.
4. Strike any vulnerable area of the body which is exposed and strike often. As you do so, move in toward the pressure of the hair pull rather than away from it.

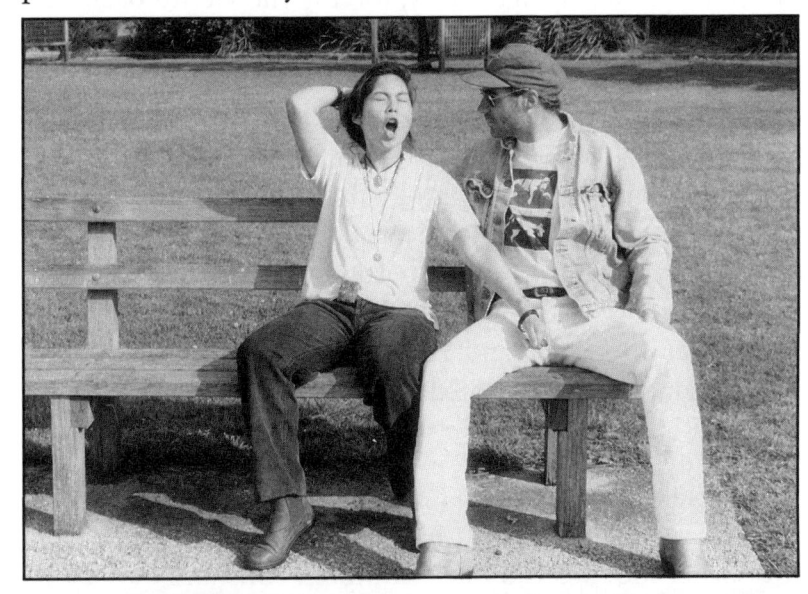

Relieve pressure on your head and hurt him in a vulnerable area — here a groin squeeze

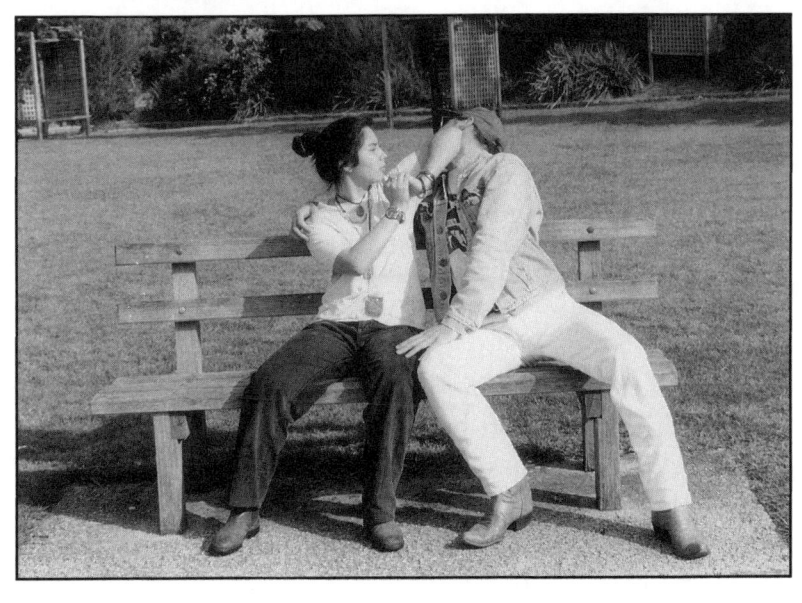

Follow through with an elbow strike

Hair pulling may be done if a man is attempting to force you to perform fellatio. It has been said that biting the penis at the base and simultaneously grabbing and twisting the scrotum cause a considerable amount of pain particularly if done with total commitment.

Here are some exercises to help you develop your understanding of balance:

Exercise 1
Have one person (the victim) stand still while the other (the grabber) circles, grabbing vigorously, forcing the victim backward (the grabber must maintain a hold so that the victim doesn't get pushed across the room). The grabs will come from the front, from the side and from behind. The grabber gradually increases the amount of force, so as to provoke fear (without causing injury). The attacker could use fear-provoking statements like, 'Keep quiet, you bitch'. The more you duplicate a real fear-producing situation and learn to function within it, the better equipped you will be to handle it if it ever actually happens. The victim must respond by adjusting her feet only and remaining emotionally centred. Practice being grabbed while seated also.

Exercise 2
Your partner grabs you with two hands and tries to grapple you to the ground. You must plant your foot in between her two feet and move your other foot around like a compass, constantly adjusting it to avoid being thrown to the ground, and adjust to the direction of the external force. If they try to trip you, you must lift your foot up quickly and plant it again.

Exercise 3
Do the same as in Exercise 2, only the victim must keep her eyes closed as she's being grabbed. (This sharpens reflexive reactions to the unexpected.)

Exercise 4
One partner will now grab the other as realistically as possible, trying to throw the victim off balance, duplicating all previously mentioned holds (as well as making up a few of your own). Restrict yourself to front-on holds for the moment. The victim will respond with appropriate techniques and strikes, as well as by adjusting and maintaining her balance.

These exercises are merely the basic building blocks to self-defence. Using them as a foundation, a firm launching pad, you can go on to devise, create, and invent your own individual responses and strategies. The more you can learn to think for yourself the more this book will help you. Ultimately the responsibility for using these techniques effectively will be yours, because, believe me, if you are ever attacked it will be the loneliest moment of your life, with only yourself to depend on.

Gradually infuse more and more realism into the holds and the resistances, including screaming, moving, striking vulnerable areas (without actually making contact with your training partner).

Exercise 5

This time practise responding to a mock attack after you have had your eyes closed. Open them as soon as your partner grabs you.

A word of warning to attackers: It's best to keep a good arm's-length away from the woman you are attacking, because if you come in too close (which I know would be a more realistic approach), you may find yourself with an elbow in the face, particularly when people start to swing around in a forward tap motion and forget to open their eyes. We have had a few bloody noses as a result of this.

chapter 4

Attacks from behind

Being attacked from behind is much more scary than being attacked from the front because there is a stronger element of being caught off-guard and of lacking control. This sort of attack is more likely to be a blitz-attack from a stranger or strangers. With someone you know it is the face-to-face build-up that is more likely to occur, but this is not a hard and fast rule.

Being lifted off the ground
This would aggravate the sense of being powerless and of being out of control, because we derive a lot of power and security from our contact with the earth (see Exercise 1 below). In this situation we must sharpen our wits and use skills that don't need grounding and are aimed backwards towards the assailant. Such tactics include the back-kick to the shins, knees and groin; the head-butt backward with the back of your head; squeezing and striking the scrotum; pulling back any fingers that are accessible; thinking heavy and continuing to resist and move in every conceivable way by keeping up the pace of resistance and being persistent; using your legs as anchors, so that the attacker has to pry you off furniture and through doorways. (It will be very difficult for a single attacker to pry your legs free from a heavy object or to stop you from hooking your legs over something at the same time as he is attempting to gag you with a hand, restrain both of your thrashing, threatening arms, as well as your butting head, all intent on donging him on the nose or doing him some other damage while he is dodging a pair of kicking heels and a gripping, squirming, resisting body.) The important thing in this situation is not to be frightened by being airborne.

If you are being pushed into a wall, get your feet up so that they hit the wall as a buffer before the rest of you does. This then enables you to give yourself a push-off. This continual resistance can also make it hard for someone to get you through a doorway. If this doesn't work, you can always play possum to regain your energy and wait for a better moment.

If you still have your feet on the ground you can use them for balance and stability. To be prepared for someone suddenly using their body weight to knock you forwards, adopt a wide stance, drop your centre of gravity and breathe out loudly if the other person's body weight hits you heavily from behind.

It is impossible to cover every way that someone could grab you from behind, but let's analyse a few in order to discover some basic principles which could be used in other problematic situations (see Exercise 2 below).

Let's first consider the mugger's hold which is statistically one of the most common ways you could be grabbed from behind. There are a number of alternative effective responses to be taken against this sort of hold, and I've found that people mostly combine three methods.

The mugger's hold

Someone grabs you around the neck with their arm and has your arm pulled back behind you, or has their arm around your neck and is pulling you backwards.

Alternative 1
1. Turn your chin toward the crease of the elbow of the attacker's arm.
2. Foot stomp.
3. Using one or both of your hands to pull down on the attacker's arm, drop your total body weight to force the clasping arm down.
4. Once he is committed to supporting your dead weight, quickly stand up and stick your chin into the space made by him accommodating your body weight, so if he resumes the choking position he will be choking your jaw, not your throat. As a bonus, this technique may enable you to head-butt as you stand up quickly, catching the assailant off guard. It also may enable you to sink your teeth into the attacker's arm, strongly encouraging him to let go of you.

The primary purpose of this first technique is to relieve the choking, because the scariest thing about this hold is the fact that you may not be able to breathe and may pass out. This hold really plays on your fear of death, particularly if accompanied by threats like 'Keep quiet or I'll kill you'.

After regaining your air supply, you can then go on to:

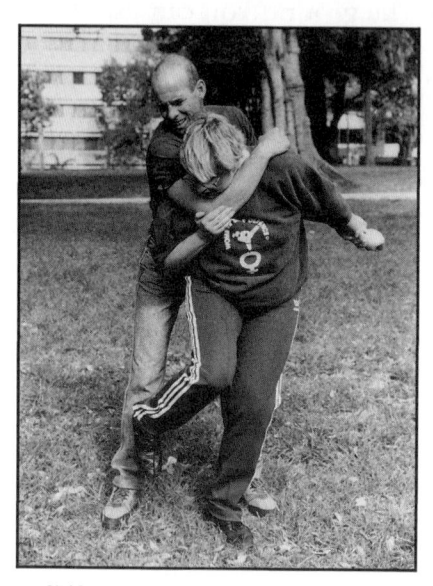

STOMP. Secure your airways and inflict pain

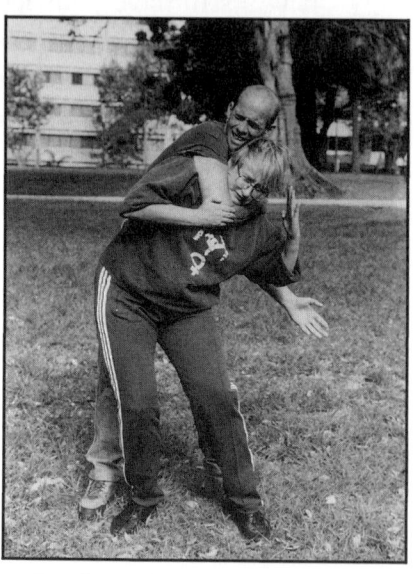

FLICK. Drop your elbow to the outside of the arm restraining your arm

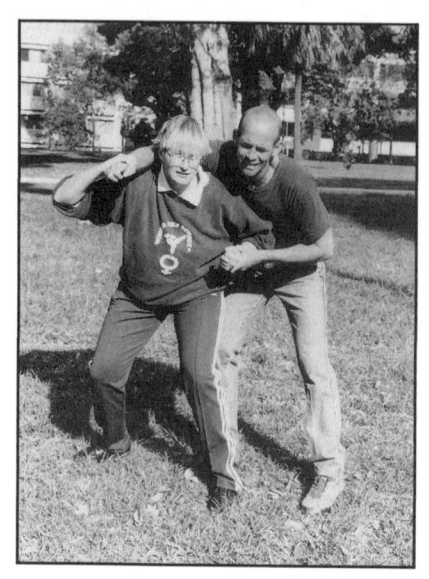

STEP. Move the foot that corresponds to the arm that is choking you behind your other foot. Turn sharply to face your attacker

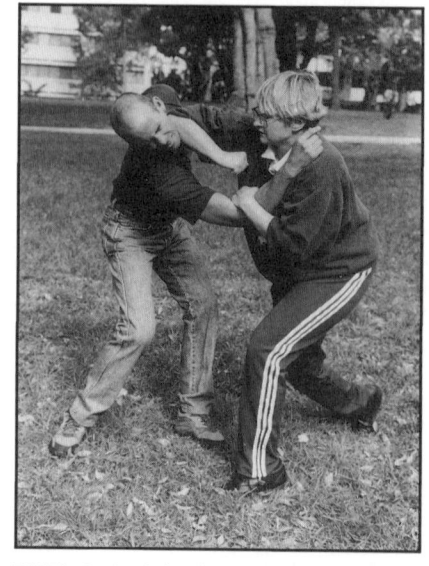

HIT. Swivel back and elbow strike your attacker, holding onto his arm and lowering your centre of gravity to pull him down

Alternative 2: Stomp, flick, step, hit
1. Put your chin down toward the crook of the elbow.
2. Inflict pain, for example, groin grab, foot stomp.
3. Place your foot that corresponds to the elbow of the attacker's choking arm behind the other foot, forming an X-shape with your legs crossed over, then turn rapidly toward the attacker's elbow, inward to face your attacker, thus again relieving the choke, and loosening the choke-hold. You can then strike to the eyes, throat, groin or *turn the tap on, and turn it off*.

If you are being held by the other arm below the elbow, you can sharply drop the elbow and shoulder down to the outside of his arm as you fan your arm upward. I usually do this to a drill of *stomp, flick, step, hit*.

The only difficulty with this technique is if your attacker has a beer gut (a malady common in Australia), which makes it difficult to rotate out of the hold. This technique is actually more difficult if the person is shorter than you because they tend to catch your balance more, pulling you into more of a back-bend position.

Alternative 3
The third alternative is grabbing the attacker's hair:
1. Grab the crown of their hair firmly (this gives you more solid leverage).
2. With a semi-circular motion pull the person around to face you.
3. Assume a wide stance to balance yourself.
4. Turn the foot and knee of the foot corresponding to the arm that's pulling the hair toward your other foot as you drop downward while swiftly jerking the attacker's hair so that the knuckles of your gripping hand are going to swoop in an arc-like motion to touch the opposite foot. You should concentrate on dropping your knee inward and keeping your body as upright as possible, because if you bend from the waist you will tend to overbalance and fall on top of your assailant. If your assailant is bald, instead of grabbing their hair, grab their neck and dig your fingers into the tendons in the soft part and then yank. Come down onto your knee if balance is a problem.

I was teaching this technique in a government department. One of my students advised me that she had a weakness in her arms due to having polio as a child. After her third lesson her

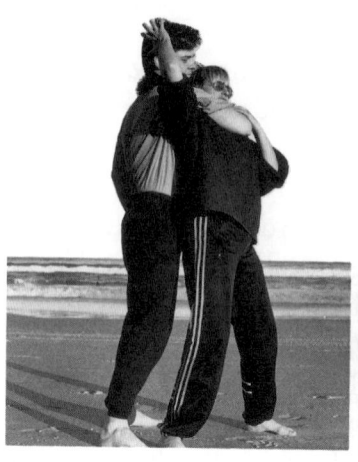

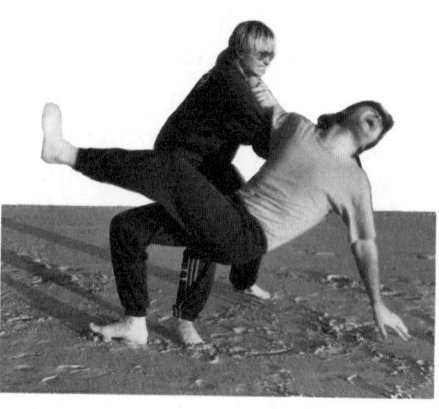

Left: *Grab his hair (or dig your nails into his neck tendons if he is bald).* Right: *Place your feet at least two shoulder-widths apart. Turn your foot and knee in the direction that you are pulling the hair of your attacker. Swoop downward in an arc-like motion so he ends up on the ground near your stable foot. Your knee can also come to rest on the ground for more stability, if needed*

(Photographs courtesy of Sandy Edwards)

teenage son, who towered over her, asked her to practise some of her newly acquired self-defence skills. He grabbed her in the mugger's hold, whereupon she promptly grabbed his hair and threw him to the ground! (This technique is more of a trip than a throw.) He had been studying karate and complained that the technique was 'not fair'. The same woman later told me that she felt that her power relationship within her family had escalated enormously since doing my course. Of course if the attacker is bald you'd better move onto the next alternative. And if they are short, fat and bald you are in real trouble!

A warning – be careful when you are practising this technique. Do it slowly rather than at a realistic speed, because if the 'attacker' is resisting falling and you are committed to topple them then the poor substitute attacker can end up with a jarred neck.

Alternative 4
This is the simplest and is generally applicable for any attack from behind. As soon as you are grabbed:
1. Stomp on the foot.
2. Grab your arm that's being held.
3. Make the hand of this arm into a fist.

4. Grab the fist, move your hips and ram your elbow as hard as you can into the solar plexus, groin or any exposed part of his body. Pull the arm away with both hands and run.

A smallish woman in a workshop used this technique, accidentally harder than she intended to, on another woman and cracked a couple of her ribs, so don't underestimate your power!

Choke-hold from behind

If someone grabs you in a choke-hold from behind you can:
1. Cross one foot behind the other in an X-like position.
2. Lift up the elbow that corresponds with the back foot as high as possible with your shoulder brushing your ear.
3. Once your foot is planted behind, you turn swinging your elbow over, following through with the other elbow in a turn-the-tap-on, turn-the-tap-off motion. This technique again enlists the power of the ground and of your torso. I have found that if the attacker moves in close to you, you will tend to dong them on the head with your elbow as you turn. (If practising, 'attackers' please remember to attack with straight arms, so as not to cop a flailing elbow in the face.)

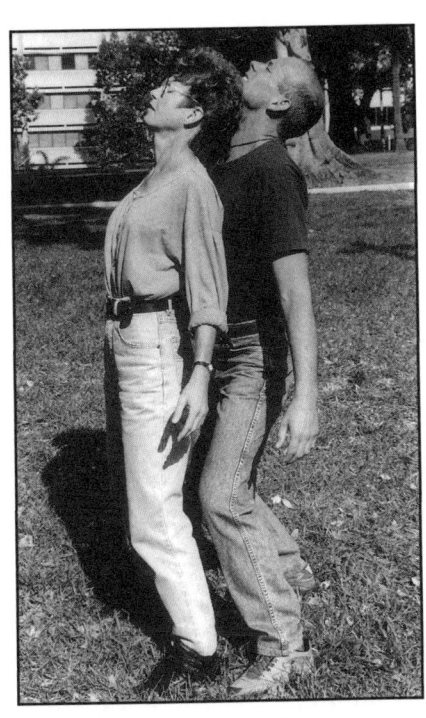

Head-butt back to his nose or chin; this is useful to release a grip from behind

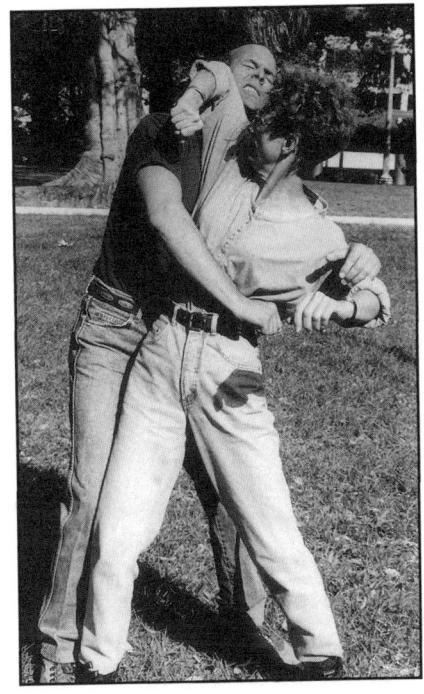

If your arms aren't restricted, you can elbow strike behind to the face

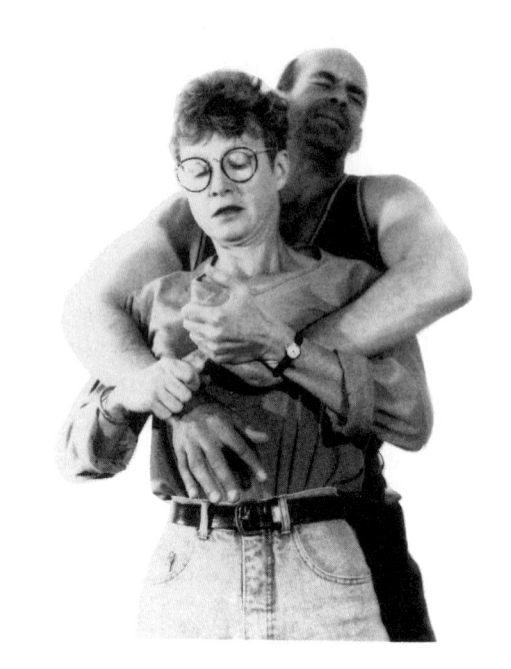

If you have access to a little finger, pull it back towards the attacker's outer forearm as hard as possible. This is surprisingly painful

Remember, the wider and lower the stance the more stable you will be. The least this movement will do is break the attacker's grip. If you are being held by the upper arms you can't circularise the technique, so you must use your straight-line techniques like back-kick, head-butt, backwards elbow-thrust.

Bearhug
This hold makes you feel like you are being squashed. Hopefully it won't happen on a full stomach! Bring your arms immediately up in front of you so that your air supply is not cut off.

Again, displace the hips in order to get a swing at the centre-line in the groin, then grab, elbow or flick-kick with the heel to the groin or stomp on the shin, foot, and head-butt backward to the nose. The tighter the arms are held the more restricted you will be in terms of grabbing, gaining mobility and delivering elbow strikes.

Arm lock
I am often asked about how to get out of an arm lock. This is a strategy that's worth a go, but you should first allow them to think that they have the upper hand before making any sudden moves. Then:
1. Take a giant step forward, straightening the arm — unravelling the lock — in a downward, diagonal direction.

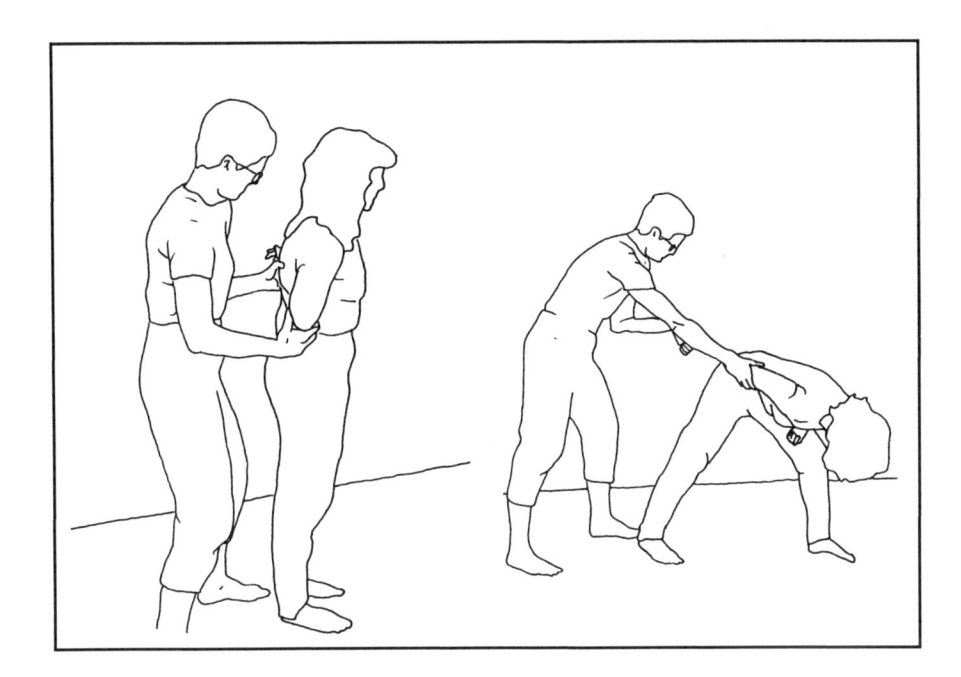

2. Then move your elbow toward your body, as you flick your hand out as if blocking, simultaneously turning to face your attacker, and following up with multiple strikes.

I had a woman in a class at a university who was held in a friendly armlock by a male friend who didn't know that the arm in question had been damaged in a car accident. She was in so much pain that she reached around and grabbed his scrotum and squeezed so hard that she ruptured both of them. For your self-defence homework, get two squash balls and squeeze them when you are watching television.

As you can see, whether you are attacked from behind or from the front or sides, the essential principles are the same. You must resist vigorously, persistently, and on all levels (that is, with all parts of your body). The more energetic are your strikes, the higher the level of your resistance, and the more you move around, the harder it is to successfully immobilise you.

The following exercises will help you to practise the techniques you'll need to defend yourself against the holds and locks described in this chapter.

Exercises
1. One partner lifts the other one up and carries her across the room. Reverse roles. One partner bear hugs the other and drags her across the room without lifting her.

Discuss how each of you felt about being up in the air as opposed to being on the ground.

2. One partner grabs the other from behind in as many ways as can be imagined and managed. Together work out possible escape strategies, both physical and psychological. Reverse roles.

3. Do the same attacking exercise, but with resistance and momentum — striking backward rapidly and strongly twenty times in various ways while screaming and resisting. Reverse roles.

4. Practise the mugger's hold on each other with increasing amounts of severity and suddenness, while the victim has her eyes shut. The attacker should be trying to elicit a fear response as well as knocking the victim off-balance. You should have red marks on your neck. If you don't, you're not being fair dinkum. Remember, the rougher you can take it and give it, the more realistic the practice (within reasonable limits), the more equipped you will be if it actually happens.

5. Practise grabbing each other in a bear hug, using your body to try and wind the other person by suddenly propelling her forward (start it softly and work your way up). Reverse roles.

Give feedback on how each level of severity makes you feel. Discuss where you store your fear in these situations and try breathing a positive light into these areas of your body as you do these exercises. It is only natural to experience fear in the midst of a 'strangling'.

SUMMARY
- **Strike vital areas.**
- **Maintain a persistent momentum.**
- **Keep striking until you are free.**
- **Keep your chin down if being choked.**
- **As soon as possible, RUN.**

chapter 5

Down, but not out: *Fighting back from the ground*

This chapter is about what to do once you are on the ground, no matter how you got there.

Avoid ending up on the ground at all costs because, let's face it, this places your attacker much closer to his objective. So once on the ground you have to fight back even stronger than before because there's often more to fight off (e.g. total body-weight pressure). But you're not licked yet, not if you are versatile in how you use your weapons and strategies.

Falling safely is a very important skill which has a broad range of applications and will be useful to you next time you stumble on the stairs, trip over something, or fall off your bike. We are going to learn a method of falling that is modified for practice in the home. Most likely an attacker will try to wrestle you to the ground by restraining your arms, so this is where your big problems will lie.

The most important thing to remember when you are falling is to disperse the impact over the greatest surface area available as you land. Try to prevent your falling weight from crushing down on any one part of your body. Ensure that your head is not thrown back towards the ground, and that no wrist, knee or elbow is in such a position as to receive the full impact of your body landing. Otherwise you stand a fair chance of breaking your bones.

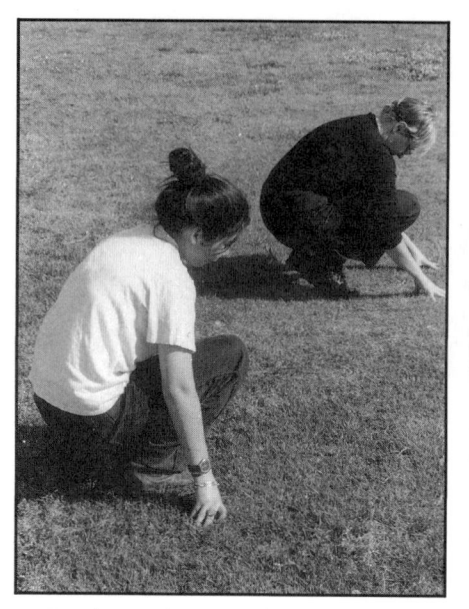

1. Bend your knees and get into a squat position
2. Keep your chin on your chest
3. Roll back in a relaxed fashion angling slightly onto your bottom and thigh (but not completely onto the side) as fluidly as possible, so your backbone doesn't touch the ground
4. Keep your knees up and your chin on your chest, slightly to the side. The extension of this movement is to roll completely over on your shoulder, but don't do this unless you have a proper padded surface beneath you. On the ground, contract yourself to make yourself as small and mobile as possible
5. Breathe out as you fall, so you don't get winded

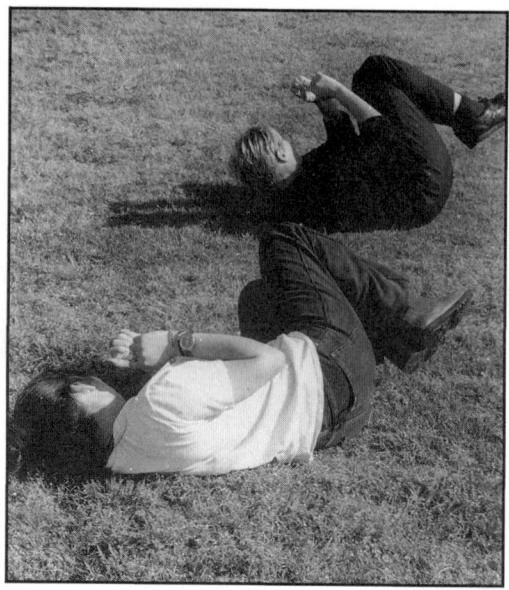

I knew one little girl who broke her fall at school with her wrist fracturing it and her collarbone simultaneously. Then there was the student who told me that she had been attacked and thrown to the ground, only later to find that she had a hairline fracture in her elbow.

Falling

I describe falling in this way rather than break-falling (which involves slapping hands and feet on the ground as you land), because I believe most women will have their hands held as they fall and the attacker's body weight will be falling on top of them, thus having the knees up acts as a buffer between the woman and the attacker's body weight. The energy of the fall should remain as fluid as flowing water. Blend with the surface; don't clash with it as you would when you deliver a punch. You should sink and relax as you fall, not try to fight it. Don't stiffen and contract.

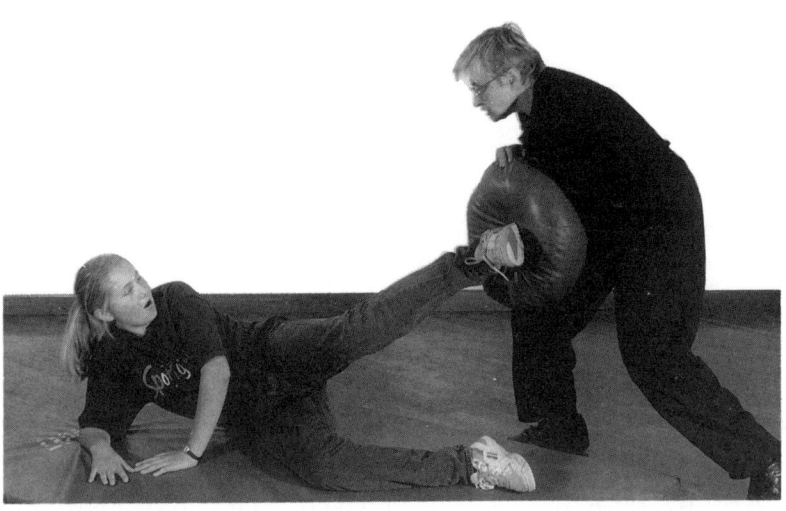

On the ground you can kick out at your attacker's accessible vulnerable points. You can also drop to the ground to this position as a defence against a punch or a weapon, or you can adopt this position if knocked to the ground. Turn your body to the side-on position and support yourself with your hands on one side of your body

During my adolescence I had a boyfriend who would go out and get intoxicated with his mates on a regular basis. He would boast to me how he would go roller skating in this condition and fall all over the place, but never get injured. I suspect it was due to his artificial state of relaxation. In Kung Fu there is a 'drunken' style, which duplicates this off-balance, relaxed state.

I recently heard of a woman who fell 5000 feet and survived with merely a few broken bones after her parachute failed to open. The explanation given was that she passed out and hit the ground in a totally relaxed state.

Break-falling from the front

Unless you have a padded surface this should only be attempted from the knees. This technique is helpful if someone is trying to ram your head into the floor or into a wall or if you are attacked from behind, since you may be pushed face down and have to break your fall.

To practise, drop to the floor from a height of only about six inches. Be sure to keep your hands spread in a triangular shape with your thumb and forefinger connected, so that the pressure goes onto your arm and open hand, down from the elbow to the tips of your extended fingers.

Dynamic techniques

These are so called because they work best if done while the attacker is still moving and committing both you and himself to a specific direction.

Grappled to the ground

In all the ground techniques it's your hips and legs which will provide your primary level of resistance, since your arms will usually be restrained and your legs are 70 per cent stronger than your arms anyway and have the advantage of being unencumbered by the need to support your body weight, as you are no longer standing.

Also with your knees up, you are now in a position, if the opportunity presents itself, to deliver a well-placed kick as your attacker comes down on top of you.

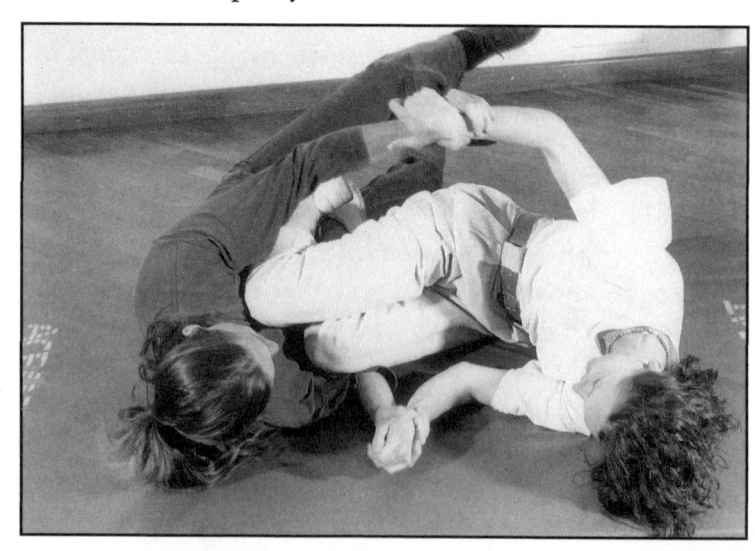

As you fall or as the person places his entire body weight on top of you, lift your legs slightly and roll your entire body to the side

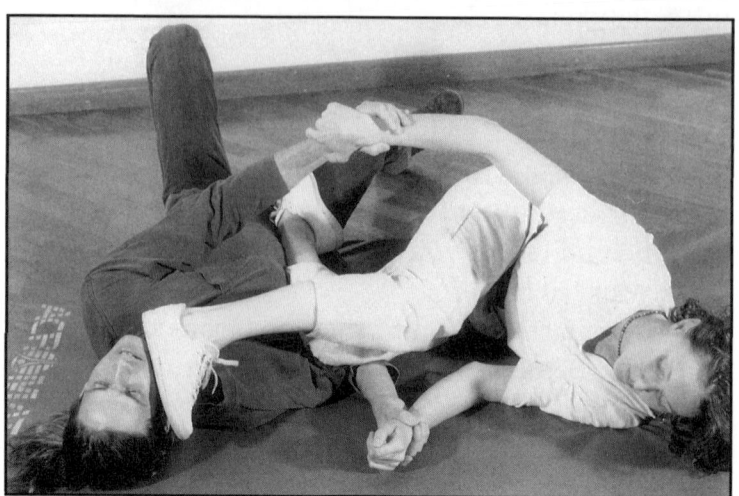

Follow through with a kick to the head

Sitting on top of you and pinning your hands

Distract – engage in conversation along the lines of 'You're too strong' or some such thing to let him think he has the upper hand. Then, the moment he relaxes a bit . . .

When practising this technique follow directions closely and provide something for your 'attacker' to fall onto, because a lightweight 'attacker' might be propelled over your head with

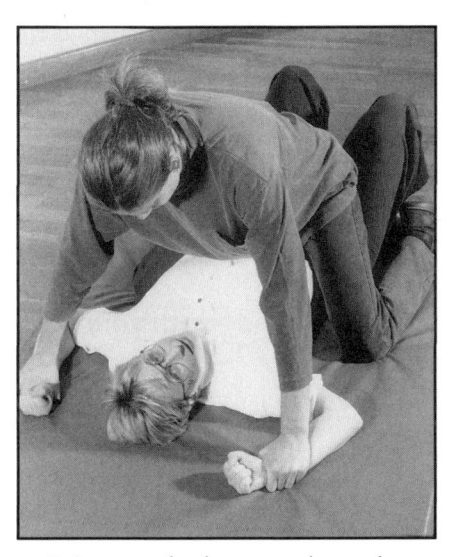

1. Bring your heels to your buttocks

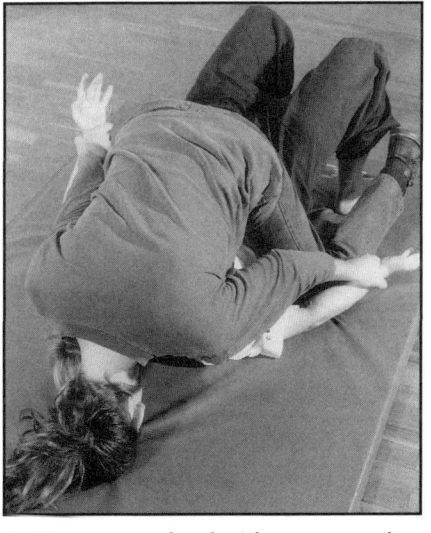

2. Turn your head sideways, so that he doesn't land on your nose. Buck your hips up very suddenly like a bucking horse, simultaneously fan your hands down, maintaining constant arm contact with the surface you are lying on. This should catapult the person forward. Grab onto the hips (if you have managed to get your hands free), arch your hips and roll him off

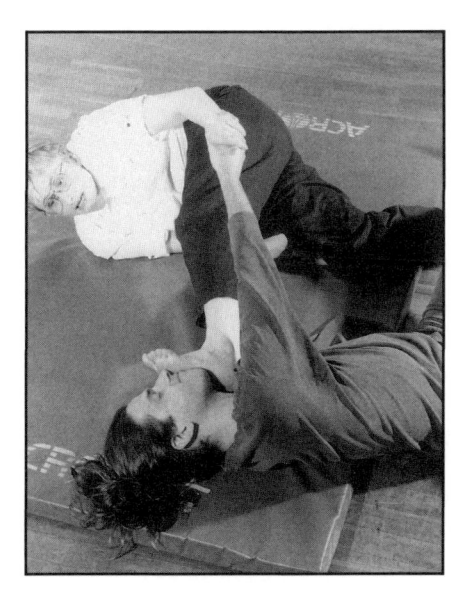

3. Always follow through with a strike. Here a kick to the face is used

unexpected speed. In classes where students have underestimated the power of this technique, there have been a couple of instances of concussion and stitches. The next technique will help to alleviate this problem.

Being choked from the ground
This will depend on the position you find yourself in, but the principle of turning the tap with your entire body motion will still apply.

1. Keep your chin down.

2. Grab a little finger. (Any finger will do, but pain will be more severe with a little finger.)

3. Strike a vulnerable area or roll your entire body with your hips and feet in an advantageous direction.

Note: Not necessarily in this order.

Attacker lying on top of you pinning your hands
Obviously in this position red lights are going to be flashing on and off in your head as your attacker is getting even closer to his objective.

1. Distract – engage in conversation or pretend to go along with it and then bite hard on his nose or top lip, or spit in his face, or jolt your arms quickly upward.

2. Let him get his legs in between yours, as this will seem like you are complying with his objectives.

Hook one leg over his leg, hooking his body to yours.
    Bring your other leg up to the side with the heel to your bum, then push up and over with the ball of your foot and thrust with your total body weight.
    Immediately knee or kick him in the head to stun him for just long enough to allow you to get up and run. It has got to be hard enough to prevent him from jumping on you again before you get away.

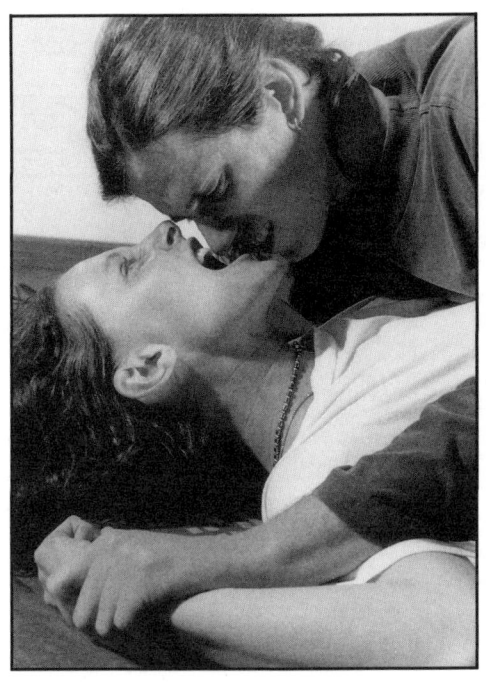

DOWN, BUT NOT OUT: FIGHTING BACK FROM THE GROUND

1. Distract — engage in conversation or pretend to go along with it and then bite hard on his nose or top lip, or spit in his face, or jolt your arms quickly upward

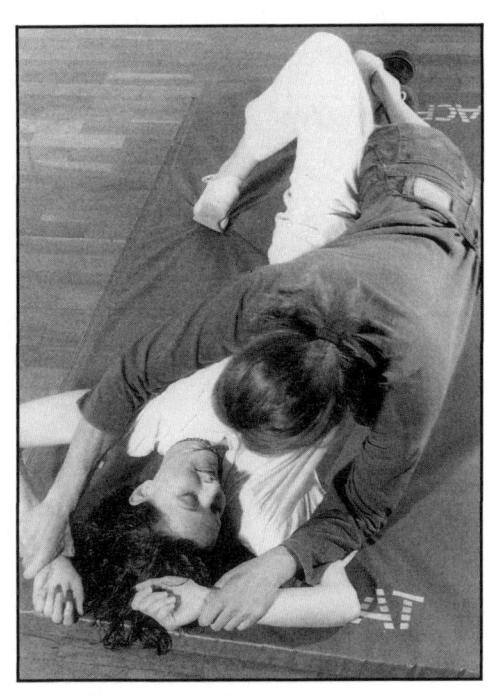

2. Let him get his legs in-between yours, as this will seem like you are complying with his objectives. Hook one leg over his leg, hooking his body to yours. Bring your other leg up to the side with the heel to your bum, then push up and over with the ball of your foot and thrust with your total body weight

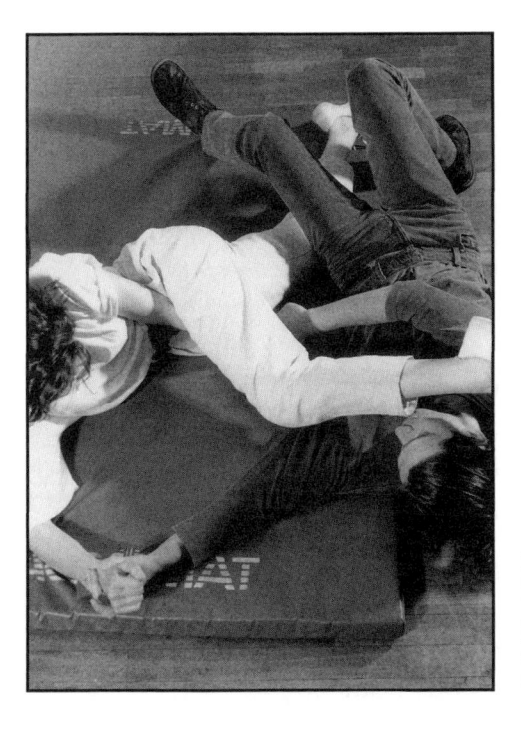

3. Immediately knee or kick him in the head to stun him for just long enough to allow you to get up and run. It has got to be hard enough to prevent him from jumping on you again before you get away

66 SELF-DEFENCE HANDBOOK FOR WOMEN

Being restrained face down
This technique relies heavily on inflicting pain before you move.

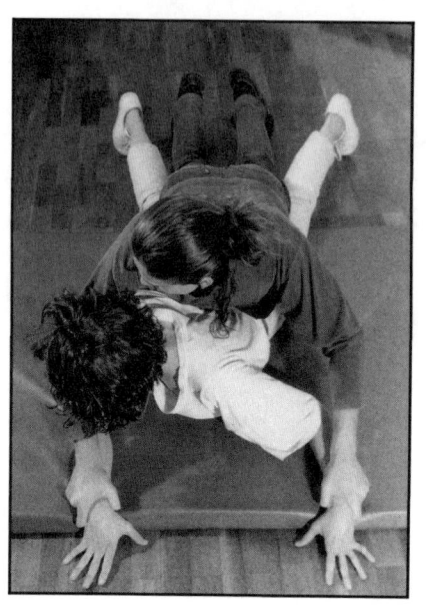

1. Quickly head-butt backward and bite his arm very hard

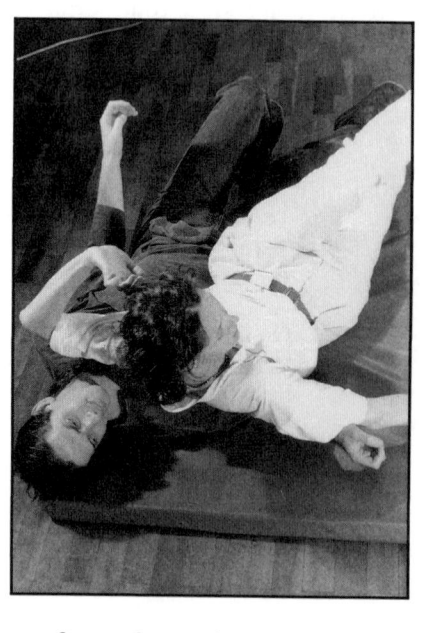

2. Slide your hands until they are up under your shoulders
3. Bring your foot up to the side as much as your flexibility will allow
4. Push up from the ground with the ball of your foot, as you simultaneously push off with the corresponding hand

5. Push the person over and hit him in the face with your elbow as you get up to flee

Defence from the side-on position
This is useful if someone is lying on top of you and your body is side-on. Possibly you are in this position because you have tried to roll him off and it hasn't worked. As the attacker is committing his body weight to one side of your body you:

1. Straighten your knees.
2. Roll towards the pressure (i.e. toward the ground) and keep rolling quickly until he is knocked off of you. Simultaneously deal him an elbow in the face.

I watched one of my students practise this technique at one of our man-attack days. The attacker was an ex-footballer standing six feet four inches and weighing seventeen stone. She used this technique to great effect, rotating continually until he went flying over the top of her slightly proportioned body.

Being kicked while you are on the ground
If someone is trying to kick you: Don't roll away from them. Roll toward their legs, grabbing hold of their legs and pretending you are a steamroller. Keep rolling toward them until they fall over or, at the very least, can't kick you any more. (Bear in mind that a kick in the head from a standing person can be fatal.)

These are only a few rudimentary positions for you to consider. Remember these basic points for ground-based self-defence:
1. Start with a distraction.
2. Use your hands as feet.
3. Make yourself as compact as possible.
4. Keep moving.
5. Strike from the ground.
6. Be fluid.
7. Keep up your striking and resistance momentum.
8. Yell 'No'.

Exercise 1
Learning to fall:
1. First practise from a crouching position.
2. Practise from a standing position by first bending your knees, then rolling.
3. If you and your partner have access to a padded surface to practise on, take turns pushing one another backwards from a standing position. (Padding may be cushions or gym mats.)

Exercise 2
Practise as full a range of self-defence techniques outlined in this chapter as possible while your partner:
1. Grapples you to the ground.
2. Attacks you from a side-on position.

3. Sits on top of you, pinning down your hands.
4. Lies on top of you.
5. Attempts to choke you from a position on the ground.
6. Restrains you face-down.
7. Kicks you while you are on the ground.
8. Sits on top of you with knees on your biceps.

Exchange roles and thoughts on which techniques you felt were more effective. Discuss ways to improve the techniques.

Exercise 3
Practising this exercise will enable you to strike whilst in a horizontal position. One partner grabs and tries to overpower the other. With her knees up, the victim rapidly strikes twenty times with her hands and feet with equal force at target areas. (See diagram of vulnerable points in Chapter 2.) Don't actually hit your partner. Reverse roles.

Exercise 4
I call this one 'World Championship Wrestling'. In this exercise your attacker seriously tries to restrain you, but it's all done on the ground. No standing up is allowed. You have to combine striking, rolling and bucking strategies, and preferably include a few dirty tricks of your own. (Biting and scratching are good ones.) You can scream also. A technique some of my students find useful is to simulate noises like those ones featured in the old Batman TV series: BAM! POW! SWOOSH!

Again make sure that you find a soft surface away from any sharp edges. Set yourself a time limit, as you will find this exercise exhausting. In class I find that this is where women usually have the most fun, often getting quite hysterical. This exercise seems to tap into a recklessness and abandon that most of us haven't experienced since childhood, if at all.

SUMMARY
- **Fall fluidly.**
- **Don't fall heavily on any one part of yourself.**
- **Strike from the ground.**
- **Hit to stun, even if you have started getting free.**
- **Use your feet as hands.**
- **Be sneaky if you are not in a good position.**
- **Distract and feign weakness until you see an opening.**

chapter 6

Blocking techniques for punches and weapons

You are more likely to be punched by someone that you know than by someone that you don't know. This is because there is usually some build-up before the punch is delivered rather than it coming out of the blue as spontaneous action. This section is particularly relevant therefore in dealing with domestic violence. If someone is angry with you they are most likely going to try to punch you in the face in a slightly circularised motion. Usually there are clear early warning signals that someone is going to punch you, things like a red face, a loud and argumentative voice, obvious anger, alcohol intoxication. In these instances it would be advisable to get out fast.

X-block
To form an X-block, move your hands into an 'X' position from your chest straight out, so that your arms connect with the punch at a 150-170 degree angle at the elbow. Let the X-block meet the punch rather than the punch meet the X-block, ensuring that you contract your arm muscles sharply as you would do in a strike when your arms connect with the assailant's punch.

Blitz attacks
The X-block is effective if someone is throwing a single technique or is slow to come out with the next blow. If someone is blitzing you with blows, as happens when you are being beaten up, grab

Bring your arms up in an 'X' position. Extend them to meet the punch with your arms at about an angle of 170° extension. The energy of the block is forward, and you contract your muscles sharply on connection with the punch. Angle upward if blocking a punch to the head

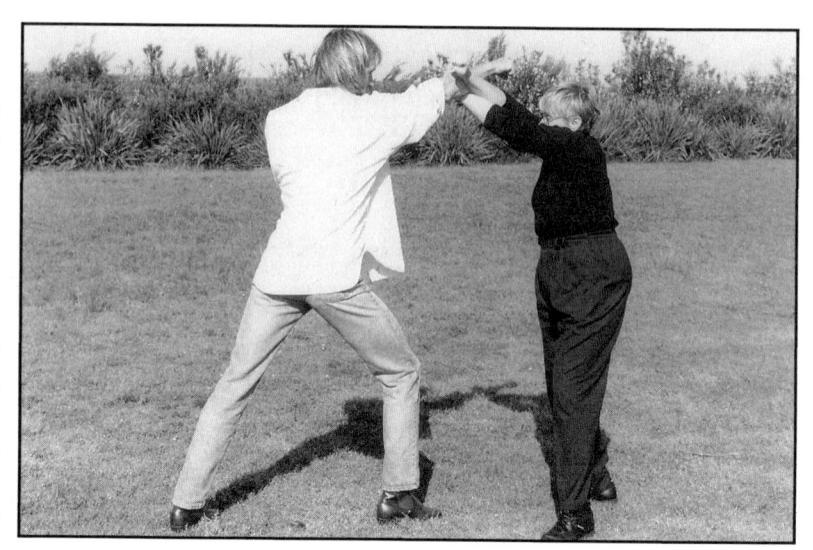

something from your environment to use as a 'shield' and then something to use as a 'sword'. If someone is bombarding you with punches, even if you receive only indirect blows to your arms you will still get an enormous shock if you are not used to being hit with forceful blows.

If you are hit on the head you may suffer concussion afterwards or at least have a headache. When you cover up like this you will get more blows on your head than on your face (see Exercise 7 below).

Having fought full contact I am very aware of what it's like to be hit and, if you are not used to it, it can send you into shock, so this exercise is like gently developing an understanding of being hit which I have developed the hard way. Don't buy into a fight if you can get away. It's very easy to get a broken nose or one of your teeth knocked out. This is why I emphasise guarding your centre line so that if you get hit it's on the side of the head. The other thing which would concern most women more than the pain is the cosmetic damage a bashing may cause.

> BLOCKING PUNCHES SUMMARY
> Move out of range. Tune into your early warning signs. Use your arms as a shield. Evade, move, block. Counter strike and move in. If need be, drop to the ground and kick the knee (or any target that is in reach). Find objects to act as equalisers (shields). Focus strikes on vulnerable areas. Don't stick around – get out of there.

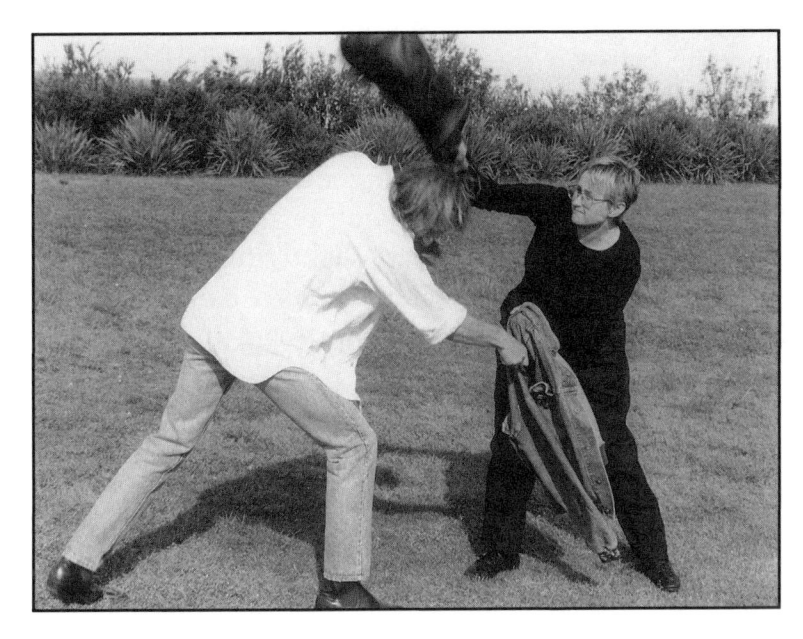

If you are attacked with a sharp weapon, you should put an object ('a shield') between you and the attacker and use another object to strike him with ('a sword')

Block and counter

If you can't find a 'shield' and you can't run away:

1. Contract yourself into a hunchback-like position with your arms around you, tucking in your elbows, facing the ground and keep moving away from your attacker and don't get cornered against a wall. (These are basic boxing principles. If you want to see how it's done watch a few boxing matches when someone is blitzing with punches up close.)

2. Move forward striking with your knee or front kick, side kick or any kick repeatedly, but don't drop your hands away from your face. Lunging in with a repeatedly kicking knee can be very effective in this context. Keep up the momentum. This may provide you with the shock value to stop the tirade of punches, enabling you to make an exit. Don't stick around to go toe to toe with your attacker (See Exercise 6 below). Practising Exercise 6 will help you to keep cool in the midst of chaos and also to pick your targets, assessing where the person is open.

Knife attacks

The essential differences between being attacked by hand as opposed to being attacked with a weapon have to do with the distance separating you and the attacker, and the consequences — a knife or club usually does more damage than a fist. I do not differentiate much between the principles used in defence against weapons and those used for defence against a punch. However, I do differentiate between the degree of alertness and accuracy needed in the different approaches. Emotionally you need to be 100 per cent on the ball when dealing with a weapon attack. In Australia the likelihood is slim of being attacked or threatened with a weapon as a victim of sexual assault or domestic violence (though in this category the chances are slightly higher). When a weapon is used in cases of sexual assault it is, most commonly, the knife. Knives are used to intimidate more than to actually do physical harm.

This fact is borne out by the Bureau of Justice Statistics Special Report, 1986: where assaults involved assailants with knives, in 78 per cent of cases the knives were not used; in 12 per cent of cases there were attempted stabbings; and in only 10 per cent of cases did assailants stab their victims. (Cited in Debbie Leung, *Self-Defense: The Womanly Art of Self-Care, Intuition and Choice*, R & M Press, Washington, 1991, pp. 42-3.)

In reality your chances of meeting up with a machete-wielding psychopath with a balaclava on his head are far fewer than of being raped by an unarmed acquaintance. Remember it's people who have some knowledge of you and your movements who will be in the best position to take advantage of you when you are most vulnerable and isolated.

Knives move very fast and do not rely on physical strength for their effect. They can be used with great competence by men, women and children. If you are approached by a child with a knife, as a friend of mine was on a late-night train, you'd better take it seriously.

If you are being threatened with a knife you must open your eyes in order to really see the situation clearly rather than be blinded by fear. Being threatened is not being dead and if someone meant to kill you and came and caught you off guard, more than likely you would be dead or stabbed. We have to get a clear idea of the person's body language. Does the person seem calm or hostile? What colour is the face — is it flushed with anger and aggression, or is it pale with fear and nervousness? If it's the latter, maybe you could talk the person down. Are the eyes cold, clear and professional? Are they moving from one side to the other rapidly, indicating indecision? What tone of voice are they using? Is it nervous, or is it angry, or is it clear and decisive? (See Exercise 1 below.)

Weapons are primarily used to intimidate and coerce. Never challenge an armed assailant who is merely trying to rob you. If it's simply things they want, it's best just to hand them over. There is no use risking your life for mere objects. But if the attacker begins to move in on you, you are in trouble and you'd better do something pretty drastic. (See exercises at the end of this chapter.) In a threatening situation the time you need to draw the line firmly as to whether you should resist is if they want to take you somewhere else in a car or room or somewhere isolated. This is when you know they have more on their mind than robbery. If you are being threatened verbally by the person holding a knife to your person:

1. Flee if possible. If that is not possible, then do your best and stay out of attacking range.
2. Keep an eye on the knife hand as well as the other parts of the attacker's body which can be used as natural weapons (e.g. the fists and feet).
3. Engage in conversation, raise your hands up to shoulder level.
4. Move away from the knife.
5. When you feel your distraction has taken effect, very sharply, as if you're striking, push your open hand half-way between the elbow and the wrist of the attacking hand. Make this movement very rapid as if you are trying to kill a mosquito on your attacker's arm. As the heel of your palm reaches the arm, close your fingers around the arm in a vice-like grip, simultaneously pushing it away. This is to make sure that you have a grip on the knife arm so you don't miss and so that your hand doesn't slide onto the blade.
6. As you do this, swivel your body away from the direction that your arm has moved, so that you are creating as much distance between you and the attacker as possible. Moving your body out of the way is very important because if your opponent is very strong you may not be able to move his arm very much. (See Exercise 2 below.)
7. As you do this simultaneously strike the attacker. All these movements must be done with the energy and commitment to shock your attacker. If you project, in any way, what you are going to do, your attacker can stop you. Swift, decisive and ruthless action is necessary.
8. You must keep hold of the knife hand while it is in range.

Other options that may be available to you after you have pushed the knife hand away:

1. Run – THE most important strategy.
2. If you can, grab something very heavy and hit your attacker with it if you have a free hand.
3. You can wait for your assailant to apply pressure on the way you are pushing (so he's pushing the knife toward you) and apply a lock.

Locks

Here is a breakdown of two locks. These must only be attempted if none of the other simpler options just mentioned are available. This is because locks are difficult things to apply when the energy of a situation is chaotic, but then again you may not have a choice. The purpose of a lock is to force a joint to go into the direction it does not want to go with the intention of inflicting pain. Because locks are certainly not a high priority, other than giving them a quick mention, I won't be going into them in great depth in this beginner's book.

Lock Number 1

X-block downward on the arm:

A knee to the groin or an elbow to the jaw wouldn't go astray at this point either. The options at this point are:
a. Break the wrist.
b. Run as soon as he hits the deck.
c. Use the assailant's weapon to further defend yourself.
d. Hit the attacker over the head with anything heavy you can get into your grasp.
e. Cut the Achilles tendons so your assailant can't chase you (find out now if you don't know where they are).

Whatever you do, it had better be fast, decisive and drastic and will change depending on the isolation and vulnerability of the situation you are in.

Lock Number 2

This is when you have push blocked to the inside of the arm.
1. Move off the line of attack ducking or evading as the attacker pushes the knife back toward you (let's assume that he is stronger than you).
2. Step beside the attacker with the knife.
3. Put the attacker's arm behind him as you rotate his knife hand upward facing the ceiling so that the shoulder, elbow and wrist are in alignment facing the ceiling.

BLOCKING TECHNIQUES FOR PUNCHES AND WEAPONS

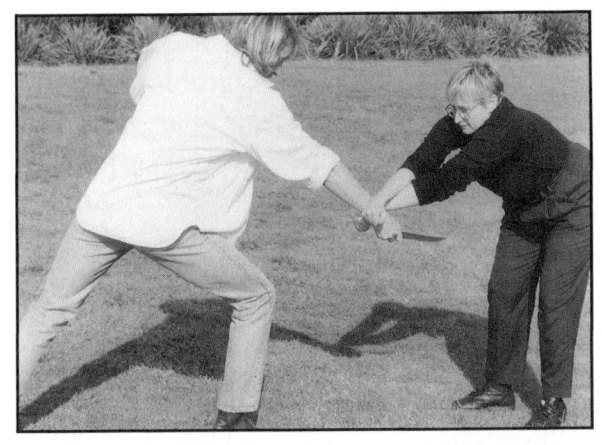

1. Make sure your attacker is pushing toward you, so you can ride his strength rather than fighting it

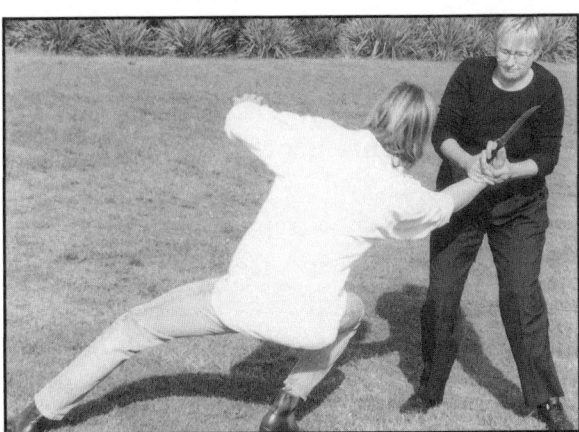

2. Make sure you are moving off the line of attack of the knife. You can do this by swerving your body out of the way and letting the knife go past you as you continue to hold the assailant's arm, providing it's going slowly enough to make this possible. Slide your blocking hand up the attacker's hand, and then with both of your hands grasp the hand that's got the knife

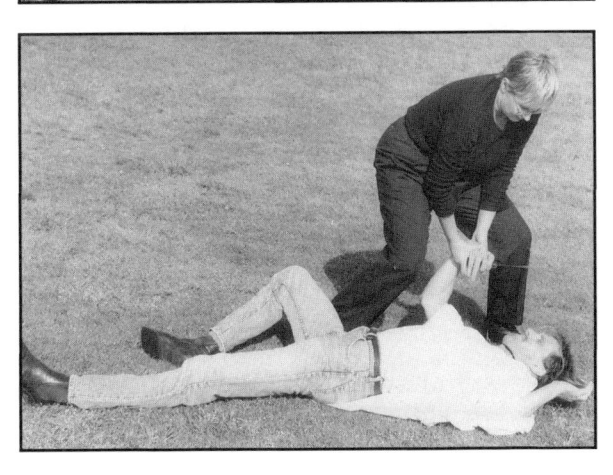

3. Push the wrist 120° toward the attacker, as if you're pushing in the cap of one of those child-proof bottles, and then turn it away from the attacker's body. Do this with the strength of your arms as well as your body, leaning into it with the intention of breaking the wrist (see Exercise 3 below)

4. Grasp the hand holding the knife with two of your hands and push it toward the attacker's elbow as you jump backwards, pulling the knife arm out as you put all the pressure of your body weight downward leaning on the shoulder.

5. His shoulder should hit the ground as all your body weight moves onto it. This has a lever effect — the attacker should move

down as you yank the hand up and simultaneously put strain on the wrist. The aim of the jump is to break the arm. After doing this, all the previously mentioned options are applicable.

BEWARE: Locks take a lot more practice than strikes. I wouldn't advise applying them in a real-life situation until you have had some expert training or unless you felt your survival depended on it and there seemed to be no other option.

A friend of mine was walking up a dark alley and was grabbed around the neck by someone holding a knife to her throat. Without thinking she elbowed her assailant in the mid-section, pushed the knife hand away and ran, jumping into a Mini Minor that had stopped at a red light. The driver reassured her with 'You'll be right luv. I'll help ya'. The success of this story lies in the woman's instantaneous reactions. It's crucial to tune into your instincts about what to do. Maybe you can talk the person down and play ball until there is a better moment – or maybe there won't be a better moment.

I am reminded of a woman at a train station who was abducted at knife point by several adolescents some of whom were female. They sexually assaulted her, then drowned her. This group had previously accosted another woman the same night who had repelled them by being verbally assertive, running away, jumping into her car and locking the doors before they had time to consolidate their attack. In the case of knife defence there must be a large emphasis on simultaneous movement at short range (Wing Chun is a style that specialises in this sort of movement).

Here is an outline of the defence:

If someone has a knife in your back:
1. Check to see it's a knife, not a finger.
2. If it's money they want, give it to them.
3. Raise your arms up so that your elbow is lower than the point of the knife.
4. Step forward and across as you swivel and connect with the knife arm in a X-blocking movement, grabbing the knife arm and striking. You must move forward as you turn and move off sideways, preferably to the outside of the knife arm.
5. Strike to the groin or other vulnerable areas or move into locks already mentioned.
6. The time you make a decision to fight for your life is if they want to take you somewhere else. At that point you know the intention is more sinister than mere robbery.

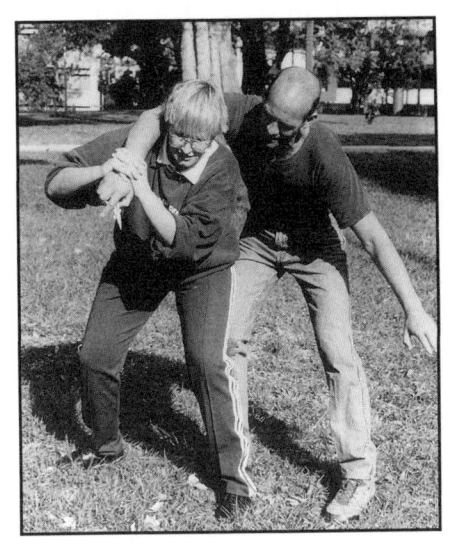

1. Reach up with your free hand and pull the knife away from you

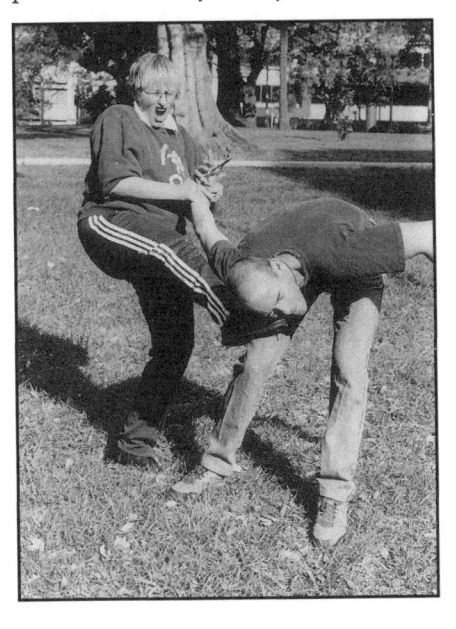

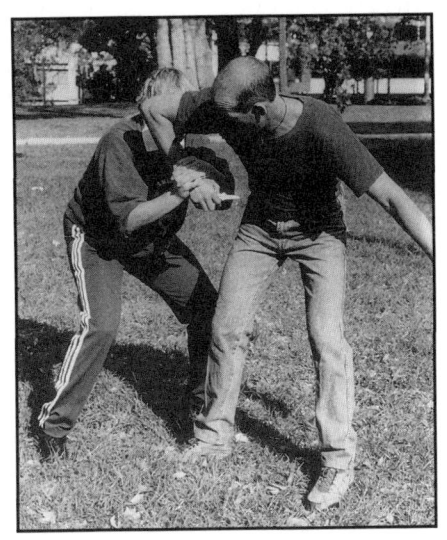

Move your hip hard into the assailant's side and elbow his mid-section, or stomp on his foot or both.

a. You can then pull the arm away and run; or

b. You can take a large step backward ducking under the restraining arm after flicking your other arm free. Grab the knife arm in your two hands and push the knife towards the attacker; or

c. Bend the wrist at a right angle to break it or to disarm him

d. If you are taller than your attacker, you should move forward rather than backward under his arm

e. Kick him in the face as you bend his wrist to ensure compliance

Dealing with a moving knife

A moving knife is estimated to travel at around 120 miles per hour, so at this stage all notions of more passive and subtle strategies must disappear because we have reached the do or die phase of escalating violence.

Our first priority besides running is to find some kind of equaliser in our environment that can be used as a shield and/or a weapon — something large, heavy or a bigger 'knife' or 'sword'. The X-block both upward and downward may be used as an effective defence against a psycho stab or an underarm thrust. I heard of a knife fight between two men. One had a knife and the other one didn't. The knifeless one picked up a piece of galvanised iron and disembowelled the other. The moral of this tale is that the person with the longer blade will get there first. I have known male martial arts experts who have come near to death when interceding empty-handed against a relatively unskilled knife-wielding opponent.

Our eyes must be wide open — so we can see everything that is going on (I think under the circumstances this might happen quite naturally) — you should be firing on all cylinders. The danger of dealing with a moving knife can't be emphasised enough. It will call for all your ruthlessness and clear-mindedness. A fact which you must accept is that if you are dealing with a moving knife you will probably get cut, but being cut is not being dead. The important thing is not to freak out at the sight of your own blood and don't look down. The moment you start to focus on your injuries you're in trouble. American studies have indicated that most stabbings and gun wounds don't actually lead to death and that some of the deaths that do occur are as much due to shock and the fear of death as being due to the wound itself. One might hypothesise that will, survival instinct and courage play a considerable part in how well you survive a wound. (See Leung, *Self-Defense, The Womanly Art...*, p. 43.)

Evasion

Evasion is the best technique to adopt because it allows you to avoid contact with the weapon or arm thrust and not receive any injury; wherever possible it should be employed. Leaving your feet planted, rotate your body sideways to avoid the downward direction of the blade. This will also work if you are stabbed in a direct straight line to the mid-section. This is true in the case of stabbing but here we must distinguish between stabbing and slashing. Evasion is the best strategy if you are quick enough. If not you are better off to block or X-block, even though it means you will get more wounds. A block will usually be more effective for a raw beginner than evasion, even though in theory evasion is superior.

Slashing

A slash can come in at any angle, so you must be alert and ready to move your body in a number of directions (see Exercise 4 below), but chiefly you must move away from the knife and stay out of range. Also at this point you don't want to commit yourself by moving before the attacker has moved, because you want to move away from the direction in which his energy is committed. Major places to avoid being slashed are the temples, underarms, inside of the thigh and the throat. Chiefly protect the organs in the chest area. If you can't avoid being stabbed in the mid-section, let it be somewhere in the lower abdominal region, so keep your head and chest covered. To fight off a knife attack effectively depends more on agility than on brute force. You need a dancer's sense of rhythm. A good rule is to never carry a weapon unless you know how to use it and are prepared to use it in your own defence, and, if it is legally required, have a license for it.

> The most important principle of defending yourself against a knife or any weapon is to use an object from your environment as a shield, such as a handbag or a chair or a waste paper basket or an umbrella and to put a large object between you and your attacker (or rather to get behind a large object). The best that you can do is put as much of everything between you and your attacker — furniture, pullovers, miles. Some self-defence teachers suggest you move a piece of clothing in a figure 8 fashion, making it harder to stab you. (It's worth a go.) Or you can wrap your jumper around your arm using it as a 'shield', but try to find a 'sword' to attack them with as well. Another option is to get something to throw in their eyes — coins, dirt, gravel, anything to blind them. I use the 'sword' and 'shield' analogy because you must pick up something to block with and something to hit with.

If you are dealing with a weapon that is essentially a large heavy object the same principles apply. You must evade the weapon and if this isn't possible you must take the blow's impact on the most dispensible part of the body (this is essentially what blocking is), so you don't get killed or knocked out (see Exercise 4, Part 6). American self-defence instructors favour dropping to the ground when confronted with a weapon and kicking towards the attacker. This removes your vital organs further from the weapon, but you will still need an offensive strategy, such as picking up a weapon or throwing dirt.

Defence against a gun

This section is not currently that relevant for residents of Australia because it's highly unusual to encounter a gunman unless it is in the context of a bank robbery, in extreme cases of domestic violence, or in the case of a lunatic on a rampage. If however you do find yourself confronted with a gun, you must assess your assailant carefully. My advice is to be very co-operative and obedient in the case of robbery. Carol Middleton in Washington DC told me of a bank robbery where everyone was told not to move. One woman turned around to ask something and was shot dead. The moral is to keep still and do exactly what you are told.

Germaine Greer tells the story of when a man drove up and pointed a shotgun at her. This was in the late 1950s as Greer was leaving a theatre in downtown Melbourne. She moved toward the car and pushed the barrel out of the way, exclaiming, 'You must be mad' and quickly exited around the front of his car, figuring that he wouldn't shoot through his own windscreen (she was right).

Running is your best weapon if the would-be assailant is in a car and you are on foot. Just be sure that you don't run in the direction the gun is aimed. In the event of someone shooting wildly — hit the deck and find cover. If they are shooting at you, run — but in an unpredictable zig-zag pattern and dive in a forward roll behind something. It's harder to hit a moving target.

Tune into your early warning signs and assess the attacker's emotional state — only resist if you are sure that they will kill you. (See Exercise 5.) Being held at gun-point, you could employ strategies similar to those used in the case of a knife attack, but more care must be taken, so I advise you first seek more expert and detailed tuition than I can offer here.

WEAPONS SUMMARY

Knife
- Stay out of range.
- Distract.
- Get an equaliser.
- Move away from the knife or move the knife away from you.
- Comply, if robbery is the only motivation.
- Act to get away and resist if they want to take you somewhere.
- Strike.
- Be sneaky.

> *Gun*
> - Comply, if robbery is the only motivation.
> - If resisting, keep away from in front of the barrel.
> - If running, zig zag in opposite direction to where the gun is pointing.
> - Find cover, if gun is shooting at you or shooting randomly. Act to get away and resist if they want to take you somewhere else.

Exercise 1: Understanding motivation

Brainstorm with each other about different emotions which would motivate a rapist (e.g. anger, hatred, aggression, insecurity, power, sadism, inadequacy, revenge, domination, desire, insensitivity, fear, peer pressure, machismo). Now do several replays with each other — one partner being the rapist and the other the potential victim. Change the motivation and the situation constantly, seeing each time how you may have to change your strategy with each new situation. If they are full-on aggressive you may try to placate them by the tone of your voice or by temporarily playing along — or you may have to take them out ruthlessly because your life's in danger. Also set the scene differently for each assault. See what sort of person would respond to being talked down and what sort of person would be inflamed by it. How quickly should you act physically in each situation? Reverse roles. Sit down and discuss your findings and what emotions you experienced as the rapist and as the potential victim.

Exercise 2

Using a piece of paper in the shape of a knife, one partner will hold the knife to the throat of the other and as soon as the victim moves the attacker will attempt to stab. The attacker will hold the knife at different angles to different parts of the body from the front. The purpose of this is to teach you to move away from the blade of the knife. It is usual for the person who acts to move faster than the person who reacts. Once you have got this done you then practise simultaneously striking at vulnerable areas, but make sure that your striking hand or knee or foot is not near the directional flow of the blade that you are pushing away, and that you don't accidentally push the blade into your own leg or arm in your haste. (With knife techniques you have to be more accurate and intentional than with bladeless defences.)

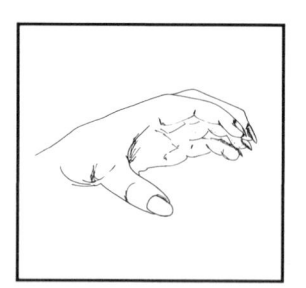

Exercise 3: Eagle claw grab

This is to practise making a connection with the hand and instantly feel the flow of the hand's direction, learning to go with it to your advantage, and then converting this into a grab. One person grabs the other one's wrist and then lets go, and the other one does it, and so on — so you have a rapidly moving flow of alternating grabs where the hand wraps right around the wrist. In reality when applying this you would dig your nails in to secure the grip, but I don't think this is advisable to do with your training partner.

Exercise 4: Evasion

1. One partner will place her foot on the other person's foot.
2. With a piece of chalk she will slash as if in slow motion so you will have time to move out of the way. She will slash at all angles moving through, so that if you don't get out of the way the chalk will mark you. This exercise starts to train your eye to see the directional flow, so you don't move toward a missile but away from it. It's also very valuable for evading punches or any missile that seems to be launched towards your head.
3. Now I want you to wait for the weapon to travel past you as you have evaded — help it by pushing it and come in with a strike.
4. Now I want you to stop the chalk before it actually comes towards you, so that you are blocking it before it has gathered momentum, and then come in with a strike. With this technique you have to either move in decisively or move out of range altogether, but don't stay in optimum range.
5. Your partner now removes her foot and she starts to slash faster, but you can have more room to move. You will have to really look outside yourself to see what is happening. This exercise teaches you not to panic and to really watch what the other person is doing and act appropriately. (Of course, reverse roles with all of these exercises.)
6. Now do all of this exercise with a rolled-up newspaper, building up to the point where if your partner doesn't get out of the way she will get a hard whack. (There's nothing like pain as a motivator.) This will help you simulate other weapons besides a knife. To simulate a punch, use an open hand so that if you do connect with your partner she will receive a slap not a knuckle sandwich.

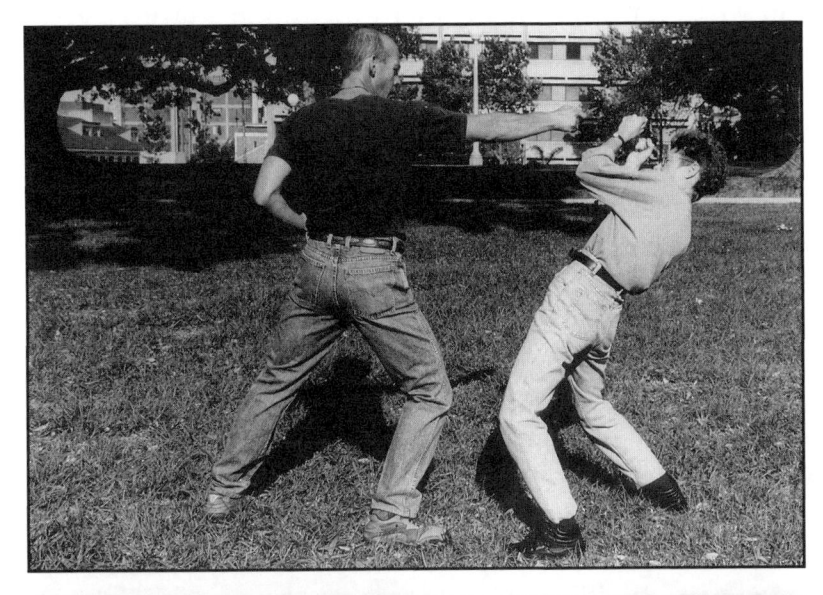

To evade a sharp weapon or punch, move away from the direction of the missile

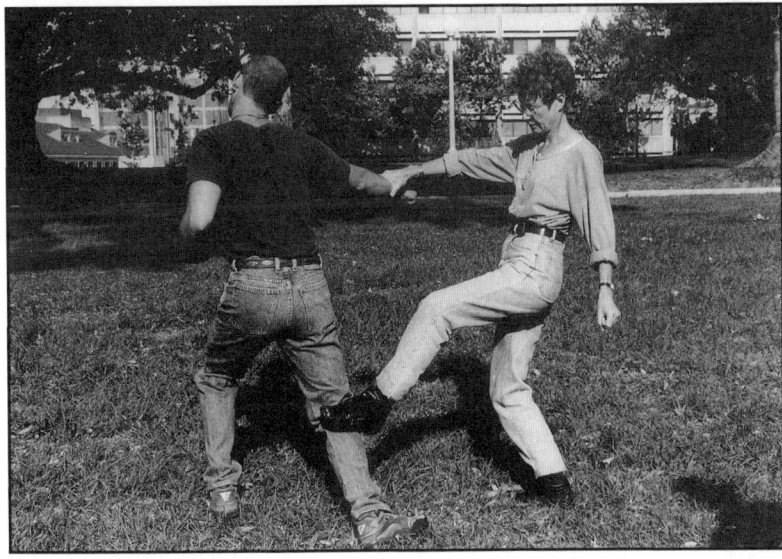

If you choose to move forward to interact with the attacker, wait for him to swing past you and push it along further in that direction whilst kicking him behind the knee or striking an accessible vulnerable target

Exercise 5: Using your environment

One partner tries to attack the other with a piece of chalk and the other must use her environment to her best advantage. Try picking up a 'sword' and a 'shield'. You can have light-weight 'swords' available, so you can really use them. You can also practise this with attacks from behind and from the side – swivelling round with a 'shield' and a 'sword'. You can practise this principle empty-handed as well – so your block is your 'shield' and your strike is your 'sword'. Also practise hiding behind furniture. Find what you could break that would make a lot of noise to attract help. Find what you could squirt or throw in the attacker's eyes. Assess your escape routes. Reverse roles.

Exercise 6: Blocking punches

1. Practise slowly blocking with an X-block, a closed fist punch — make the punch slow.
2. Now practise with an open-handed tap to the forehead as fast as you can so your partner can practise her blocking reflex. The faster you strike, the faster your partner has to block. If you miss you will only get a tap on the head, so the dynamic is the same, but the consequences and intention are different.
3. Now do the same thing with circular punches — slowly with a closed fist and fast with an open hand.
4. See Evasion Exercise 4 for evading punches.
5. Practise blitzing. Deliver rapid punches one after another, but with an open hand while your partner guards, moves and kicks simultaneously.
6. Make this a very dynamic exercise, making surprise lunge moves towards your partner's centre line. You will find if someone is out of control and striking in a circular motion usually their centre line is open. In reality you could also lunge in with a headbutt or elbow while still keeping your face guarded. If you lunge in with the knee you can grab them around the neck to balance yourself (keep strikes open-handed and use control if kicking partner, or use a kick bag).
7. Reverse roles.
8. Discuss your results and what you have learned.

Exercise 7: Tolerating blows

Your partner hits you open-handed on your head reasonably hard to give you a shock. Reverse roles. This is like a slap on the head rather than a punch. This is an optional exercise, but it will give you some idea of what you may encounter if someone is serious. Do this as forcefully as is tolerable and undamaging. Sit down and talk about how it feels to be hit and to hit back in order to cause pain. (Many women have to break through the barrier of deliberately aiming to hurt someone.)

chapter 7

Machismo:
Is there a cure?

I call machismo a 'disease' because it causes both women and men dis-ease in different ways. The Oxford English Dictionary defines machismo as 'The quality of being macho, male, virility, masculine pride . . . the essence of manliness . . .; "in prison toughness may substitute for intercourse as a measure of machismo"'. (Oxford English Dictionary, 2nd edition, vol. IX, Clarendon Press, Oxford, 1989.)

The structural and cultural environment that allows the machismo virus to incubate is based on men having power and women not. Pride and virility – the power of procreativity, capability for sexual intercourse – is seen as the cornerstone of male supremacy. The link between machismo-infected sexuality and how society operates will form the basis of this chapter.

Some symptoms of machismo you may detect from the men in your life, particularly if you try and use them as training partners, are:

1. Making absolute statements like 'You are wasting your time doing self-defence. No woman could ever defend herself against any man'.
2. Ridiculing and making jokes about your efforts to be strong.
3. Feigning extreme fear and protecting their vital male bits behind desks, chairs, filing cabinets, and other objects of furniture when you come into a room.
4. Making moronic quips like 'You do self-defence, well I'd better watch out, ho ho'. Can you imagine them saying this to a man who was learning some form of self-defence, and if not, why not?

5. Jumping out and grabbing you at inappropriate moments in what they suppose is an indefensible lock, and saying inane things like 'Now use some of your self-defence on me and see if you can get out of this'.

Don't practise with such men unless you are really prepared to let them have it, or you will be like a tigress hunting without her claws. It can be very disillusioning when you are just starting to practise newly learned techniques that seem not to be working and mainly because you are not committing your energy for fear of hurting the man involved or his fragile male ego. Usually it is best to have a female training partner initially; and if you do want to test your techniques out on a man make sure that he does not have any of the above symptoms.

What many women fail to understand about rape is that it is not so much an act of lust, but an act of personal violence fuelled by a lack of respect for 'the victim'. As sociologist, R. W. Connell, points out 'it is often difficult to see beyond individual acts of force or oppression to an overall structure of power . . . rape is routinely presented in the media as individual deviance. But most rapists are motivated by the sense of power they experience in a rape, rather than the sexual release of the act itself' (*Gender and Power*, Allen & Unwin, Sydney, 1987, p. 107).

This is a global affliction. As Naomi Wolf has reminded us in *The Beauty Myth*, the ratio of gender-based power is fixed and international. According to the Humphrey Institute of Public Affairs: 'While women represent fifty per cent of the world population, they perform nearly two-thirds of all working hours, receive only one-tenth of the world income and own less than one per cent of world property.' The report of the world conference for the United Nations Decade for Women agrees, when housework is accounted for, 'Women around the world end up working twice as many hours as men' (Naomi Wolf, *The Beauty Myth*, Vintage, London, 1990, p. 23).

The machismo virus strikes every man to a greater or lesser extent, and rape or the fear of rape is used to curtail the freedom of women. The word 'rapist' tends to conjure up images of someone like the Yorkshire Ripper who mutilates and sexually abuses women and puts whole communities in a state of seige. These are the ones with the more progressed and virulent strain of the machismo virus, but there are many strains. Those affected can be placed on a continuum or a pyramid, with the sadistic psychopath at the top and the angry, violent wife-basher in the upper to middle section, moving down to the dealers in mild sexual harassment and sexist remarks at the bottom. This harassment may be a prelude or a testing for potential victims of future severe or fatal rape attacks. 'If it happens in an alley, it's rape. If it's your date, it's love.' (See Andra Nedea and Kathleen Thompson, *Against Rape*, Farrar, Straus & Giroux, New York, 1974, p. 12.)

Too often the extent to which rape and violence are considered 'acceptable' depends on the degree to which a man has property rights over the woman he is abusing. I remember visiting a friend whose husband would verbally abuse her to humiliate her in front of her friends. In the middle of an argument he would yell, 'I own you' and she would retaliate, 'No, you don't'. He challenged, 'Who owns you then?' She had to think for a moment or so and then said uncertainly, 'Nobody does'. Historically women have had few independent rights and have been seen as property or a possession. It is only recently that raping your wife has become illegal in Australia: 'In the rape statutes of 50 US states its very definition provided that rape is the forcible penetration by a man of a woman not his wife' (*Against Rape*, p. 13). The Groth study of 1979 documented convicted rapists' attitudes and motives:

1. Anger rape (40%). The rapist intentionally means to hurt and degrade the woman and harbours a large degree of violence and hostility for her.
2. Sadistic rape (5%). The rapist enjoys torturing his victims in a premeditated fashion. 'He may stub out cigarettes on her skin, shove bottles into her anus, and push fists, sticks and rifle barrels into her vagina, carve her up with a knife or batter her to death.' (From *Face of the Rapist*, David Shapcott, Penguin, Auckland, 1988, p. 42).
3. Power Rape (55%). The rapist sees women as made for their convenience, basically as 'pieces of ass' ready for the taking. He is under the delusion that she enjoys it or he will get away with it and get kudos from it.

A common example of 'power rape' was recounted in *Face of the Rapist*. A young man discovered an unconscious woman in the back bedroom at a party. He quickly had sex with her and returned to the party. He later presented the rape to his peers as a heroic escapade (*Face of the Rapist*, p. 45).

These categories are not fixed. What about the man who regularly bruises the features of his wife, putting her in hospital, as well as sexually abusing her? I believe his motives are sadistic, anger-based and power-related. The shame and social stigma associated with being the victim of rape has meant that women often have not reported the crimes against them.

One myth that needs to be dismantled is that rapists are likely to be deviants and total strangers. More often than not the rapist is known to the victim. Date rape and acquaintance rape account for more incidences of rape than attacks by strangers. One study indicated that: 24 per cent of attacks happened in the victim's house as opposed to 2.7 per cent in an ill-lit street (see *The Rosanne Bonney Study*, Bureau of Crime, Statistics and Research, New South Wales, September 1985, p. 40). It doesn't even touch on the domestic violence and incest epidemic that operates behind the closed doors of a significant proportion of Australian homes.

It's much easier to think about the boogieman than to think about the date who just won't take no for an answer if he has spent money on you at dinner. In *Stopping Rape* a study of 832 high-school students revealed that:

- under a number of conditions which the male interpreted as being 'led on', he felt entitled to force the woman to have sex;
- between 36-45 per cent of men thought it 'OK' to force sex if the man spent a lot of money on a woman;
- forced sex was also 'OK' if the male was so 'turned on he can't stop'; if 'he knew she had sexual intercourse with other guys'; if the woman was drunk or stoned; if she let him touch her below the waist; or and if they had been dating for a long time. (See Bart and O'Brien, *Stopping Rape: Successful Survival Strategies*, Pergamon Press, 1985, p. 98.)

What woman hasn't wrestled in the back seat of a car beating off unwanted advances? Older and wiser, I now select partners who understand that 'no' means 'no'.

'Ordinary' people could perform atrocities at Buchenwald and My Lai because their victims were perceived of as 'Jews' and 'gooks'. These murderers had been told, and they believed, that the people they were killing were lesser beings, not beings with rights such as their friends and families might be expected to enjoy. (See Nedea and Thompson, *Against Rape*, p. 30.) This is the basis of the most horrible racist crimes and the most horrible sexist crimes. When I was at school one of my girlfriends told me of a young man of our mutual acquaintance who had participated in a pack rape. He was young, sensitive, attractive. He told her he went last, not really wanting to do it. Although guilt and remorse plagued this seventeen-year-old, he joined in the rape rather than risk 'losing face' in front of his friends.

Recognising that rapists can be the 'boy next-door' does not make the act less horrible. Rather, it brings into question the society in which ordinary men can rape. How do women become dehumanised in the eyes of men? Pornography is the most graphic example of this process. In hardcore pornography women are portrayed as mere bodies – mindless bits of meat to be manipulated for male sexual gratification. The soft-core variety is seen by everyone and is more damaging because it is considered 'normal'. How often do we see a semi-nude woman used to sell a car, motorbike, holiday resort or electric drill? This is in the streets, on television, accosting us and our children every day.

The uncontrollable, irrepressible nature of the male sexual urge is another myth that haunts us: 'I was just so turned on I thought I would pass out. She might have struggled but no more than women usually do. I couldn't stop myself. I wanted to see her naked, to touch her, to ram myself into her, to feel the ecstasy – it was so good'. Justification is often given in the form of 'she asked for it' or 'she deserved to be raped'. Imagine a bank robber hitting a bank manager and robbing a bank, saying 'I couldn't stop myself. He was just asking for it. I had to have it, to feel the ecstacy of spending all that money! He put up a bit of a struggle, but no more than the usual bank manager would. He really wanted me to have it or why would he have had so much money changing hands in his bank in the first place?'

In *Stopping Rape* a telephone survey of men who had committed rape and not been caught reported that, for the most part, the men felt that raping women had no negative effect on their lives or their self-image. Indeed sixteen per cent felt that having raped had enhanced their self-image and had had a positive effect on their lives. Their decision to rape was based on the potential reward (e.g. ego enhancement) and on the low probability, of serious negative consequences such as bodily injury or imprisonment (*Stopping Rape*, p. 98).

Women are often the harshest critics of other women. This is partly a defence mechanism. If you can point the finger at someone who 'deserves' to be raped and put the 'slut' tag on her, it makes you feel safer because rape only happens to 'bad' girls not to women like yourself. We have to differentiate here between being responsible and being vulnerable. Even when a woman ends up in a vulnerable position, she is never responsible for someone taking advantage of her situation. In most Australians' minds the case of Anita Cobby looms large as the most publicised gang rape-murder trial in Australian history. Anita Cobby was walking to her home from the train station in the western suburbs when she was dragged into a car, driven to a deserted place, beaten, raped and knifed to death by five men. I recall a television interview with a female friend of one of the killers who asked, 'What was she doing walking around the streets that time of night anyway?'

A lot of men feel justified in raping a woman because they genuinely believe that she enjoys it: 'But a little bit of a struggle turns everyone on. She salves her conscience, makes you a little keener and when the struggling stops you know she's ready for it' (*Face of the Rapist*, p. 17).

In addition to their own feelings, many women who have been raped face the burden of blame heaped upon them from their male partners. One case cited in *The Politics of Rape* recalled a woman who was hospitalised following a rape being asked by a male psychiatrist there: 'Haven't you really been rushing toward this very thing all your life?'. And when she returned home, her husband angrily accused her, 'If that's what you wanted, why didn't you come to me?' (*The Politics of Rape: The Victim's Perspective*, Diana E. H. Russell, Stein & Day, New York, 1975, p. 18.)

More scary to a man than being brought up on a rape charge is the threat of a woman who dares to show signs of an uncensored libido. If a woman displays a strong open and honest desire for a lot of sex, or seeks sex with a variety of partners, she is seen to be afflicted with nymphomania. A male friend complained to me about his former girlfriend who was wanting sex morning, noon and night. He couldn't handle it! The same behaviour in a male would be merely seen as 'virility'. To curb such abnormal behaviour in women labels such as 'slut', 'slag', 'whore', and 'deserve to be raped' are used.

Only second to the threat of a sexually powerful woman is the physically powerful one. The ban on women harnessing the tools of violence is a straitjacket of social conditioning. I have found full-contact tournament fighting a valuable way to gain an understanding of transcending fear and translating it to action. It's

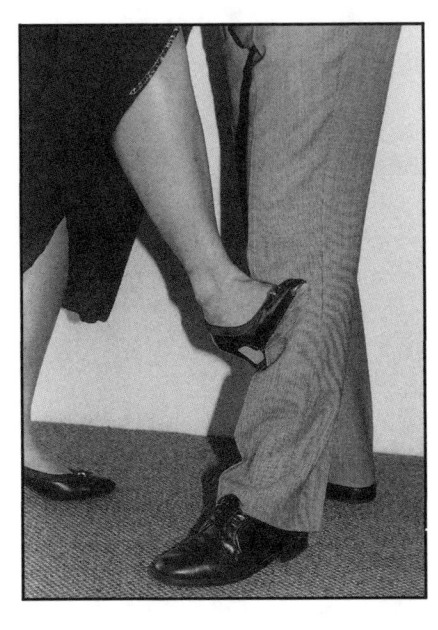

Calf scrape — even high heels can be a weapon. Here they are used close-range against an unwelcome invasion into her space

scary to jump in the ring with someone who is trying to knock your head off, but is it any more scary than being confronted by a large male who is trying to rape you? How else are we going to learn about the tools we need to defend ourselves except to put ourselves in extreme, yet at the same time, controlled situations where there are rules and padding for protection.

Yet any woman who does harness these skills is ridiculed and her femininity is brought into question. There are laws preventing women from functioning in a warrior-type fashion even today. As a kick-boxer, I was invited to participate in a women's tournament at Sydney Town Hall in 1984. The then Premier of New South Wales used the Theatre and Public Halls Act of 1908 to stop us. He publicly stated, 'Even in this age of anti-discrimination and unisex I feel the public thinks the spectacle of two women fighting each other to be degrading and totally unacceptable.' We held the tournament twice in defiance of the ban, risking fines and imprisonment, to champion the rights of women to fight publicly. We won the court battles and I received $7200 in compensation from the Human Rights Commission for being denied a service on the basis of sex.

Are men ever on the receiving end of what is dished out to women? Yes, they are. Machismo is a system that works against everybody, not just women and children. Machismo can put men out of touch with the full range of their feelings. It can also foist onto them unwanted sex/power roles. Prisons provide a

Relationship of Attacker to Victim
- 30.3% Friend/acquaintance
- 28% Stranger
- 17.1% First-time acquaintance
- 4% Driver who rapes hitchhiker
- 3.9% Stepfather
- 3.5% Estranged lover/spouse
- 3.1% Relative other than immediate family
- 2.6% Man who rapes prostitutes
- 2.2% Father
- 1.8% Neighbour
- 1.7% Brother or brother-in-law
- 0.9% Other 'trust' relationships including baby-sitter, police in charge of jail cells
- 0.9% Work associate

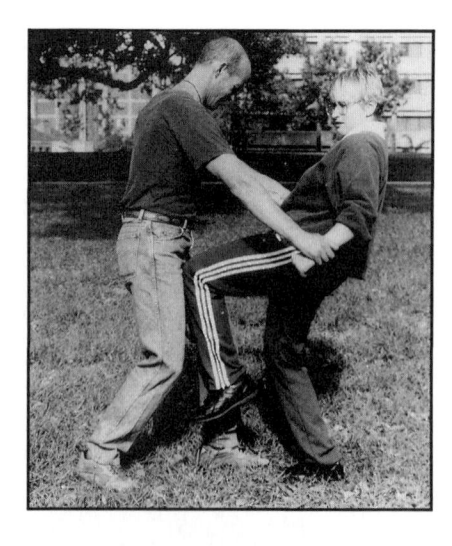

Where a Sexual Offence Occurs
- 23.7% Park/bush/deserted area
- 17.8% Vehicle
- 14% Victim's house (offender was allowed entry)
- 11.9% Offender's house
- 10.8% Victim's house (offender broke in)
- 5.3% Mutual house
- 5.3% Other house
- 2.7% Street/lane
- 2.2% Party/disco/hotel
- 1.7% More than one location
- 1% Shelter/institution
- 1% Workplace
- 1% Shopping complex
- 1% Public transport
- 0.6% Garden of house

Source: *The Rosanne Bonney Study*, Bureau of Crime, Statistics and Research, NSW, September 1985 p.40.

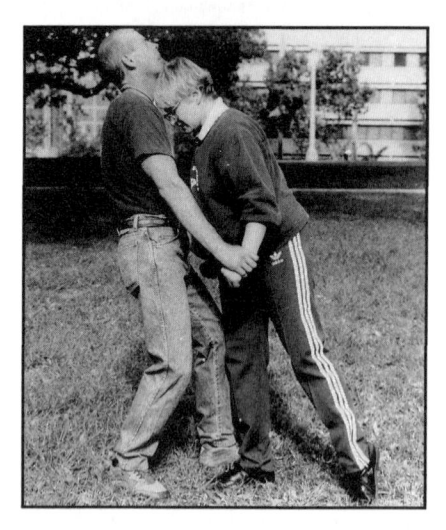

microcosm for this understanding. Here we see men who display characteristics commonly attributed to women (younger, weaker, smaller, better looking) being sexually abused by the older, tougher, uglier and bigger.

However, oppressive power relations between the sexes are not inevitable:

> There is no rape among the Arapesh studied by Margaret Mead. This small tightly knit community live in the harsh mountain regions in New Guinea. They survive in a frugal environment by depending on one another and peacefully co-operating with one another. There is no trace amongst them of the aggression and competitiveness that characterise the Western quest for survival. They do not embark on warfare, there is no kudos in being a

warrior, killing is not a sign of manhood or manliness. Indeed, men who have killed are viewed with some discomfort. (*The Facts of Rape*, Barbara Toner, Avon Books, London, 1982, p. 51.)

For the sakes of both men and women, machismo must be shown for what it is: not desirable, nor mysterious, nor powerful, but dangerous, uncivilised and brutish — and not to be tolerated. Join a women's self-defence course and see where it takes you. It may open your mind to new levels of understanding. You may find that it opens doors you never knew existed and close a few that don't add to the quality of your life. Doing a course isn't 'The Answer', but it's at least a start and may help you to start discovering some of the questions. The child protection literature on child sexual abuse has a slogan, 'No excuses, never ever'. The same slogan applies to rape. Rape is political, not sexual.

chapter 8

Domestic violence

The most ugly and insidious way the machismo virus effects the very fabric of society is in the form of domestic violence. Here we see women intimidated, bashed, raped, killed and just plain worn down. It is conservatively estimated that domestic violence is a regular feature of one in four Australian homes. According to Jocelynne Scutt, marital rape and murder and domestic violence 'would not happen without the tacit agreement of society that women are owned by men, that men have a right to push women around, to use them sexually as they choose and finally to kill them out of passion if a wife decides to leave' (*Even in the Best Homes*, Penguin, 1983, pp. 98-9).

As seen in a 1989 survey outlined in the *Domestic Violence Report of the National Committee on Violence* from the Institute of Criminology, women are 'asking for it' when they dare to transgress their allotted role of wife and mother. The survey revealed several commonly accepted legitimate reasons for a husband to beat his wife. These included arguing or refusing to obey him; nagging; refusing sex or admitting infidelity.

The general public and those in authority are often reluctant to interfere even though they may hear continuous screams for help and see women getting bashed about. Some are even reluctant to telephone the police, finding excuses for the offender's violence, such as, 'Some men have no alternative, she is lazy and she nags ... It's basically natural. Violence is instinctive to all men.' (See Jane Mayford, *National Committee on Violence – Domestic Violence No 2*, 1989, Institute of Criminology.) Susanne Hatty's recent research on attitudes towards domestic violence clearly indicates this. A female police officer who had dealt with cases of domestic violence commented on how her behaviour and attitudes had changed: 'Before I was very passive in my relationships with men. I just went along with what they wanted. Not now. I've learned to stand up for myself. I've learned that if you don't do this you're sunk.' (See Graham Williams, 'Women and Cops', *Sydney Morning Herald*, 5 July 1989, Agenda article on Susanne Hatty's new study on *Police Attitudes to Domestic Violence*.)

Reasons often given as to why women stay with violent men include that they were financially, emotionally and sexually dependent, wanted to maintain the family unit, wished to live up to certain perceived social expectations, and suffered from low self-esteem. The myth that women enjoy being bashed echoes the myth that women enjoy being raped. It's a way of displacing the responsibility and blame from the abuser to the abused so that the crime can be seen as the responsibility of the woman involved. Even a wife who fulfills all her domestic duties may find herself being used as a whipping post for her husband's pent-up frustrations, possibly caused by things outside the home, such as his work conditions.

The degree of violence that has been statistically recorded for domestic violence is far greater than for sexual assault as a whole. A self-defence course can benefit the domestic violence victim in a number of ways:

1. It can sharpen up your awareness that violence is impending, by making you more aware of early warning signs. We always advise exiting and avoiding a confrontation where possible.

2. Women in a physically abusive relationship should focus on the skills of blocking and evasion since punching, kicking, being rammed into walls and furniture, or threatened with a weapon are far more prevalent here.

3. If you are driven to the point where you must strike or do something to save your life or to stop someone causing serious harm to you or your children, then you must do it with maximum efficiency. Some will say this is like putting out the fire with gasoline. We don't advise that you learn self-defence in an effort to train to go toe to toe for fifteen rounds with an angry violent, aggressive, larger and often drunk male in an attempt to knock his block off. We advise striking if it will be effective

in distracting your assailant, so you can retreat from the situation. Some women express fear of revenge at a later date.

My answer is that extreme situations call for extreme measures. If you can't get away or get help and your life or your personal safety or that of your child is threatened, you are better off acting in your own defence with a degree of force appropriate to the situation than worrying about what your abuser may do later — there may not be any later. Action can include:

1. Using an object from your environment as a shield or as a weapon.

2. Screaming 'fire' to attract attention (your neighbours may not come if they think it's a 'domestic', but they might call the Fire Department or come to check it out). If you smash something noisily, this may attract enough attention to get people running in to inquire.

3. Running to get out of the situation.

4. Pre-planning an escape route for yourself and your children in the event of an emergency, e.g. always carry the car-keys on your person.

5. Striking a vulnerable area of your attacker's body with your body or something from your environment (with a degree of force that is justified in the situation). A self-defence course can provide these strategies, but also, more importantly, it can create a shift in confidence and self-esteem. It can stimulate the abused woman to begin a process of reassessment and review of the general quality of her life; it can then prompt her to begin thinking seriously and constructively about the decisions she may need to make to set about changing her situation. In the early stages of deciding to leave a violent relationship, self-defence can be a way of moving the woman from the victim position. Participating in this sort of activity helps her to deal with pent-up emotions, encourages her self-determination and a healthy self-centredness. This will aid in changing her outlook and reaffirm the value of quality in her life and her relationships, so that she will not easily be attracted back into another violent and abusive relationship. At this time of uncertainty and transition in their lives, women need to draw on every resource possible to keep them feeling positive and directed.

Domestic violence has been described as functioning in a repetitive cycle where there is:

1. A build-up of tension (arguments or alternatively a silence that screams);
2. physical abuse (violent episode), followed by
3. the honeymoon period – the abuser is remorseful and on his best behaviour (Prince Charming);
4. and then the tension starts again. The cycle can go on for a lifetime. Generally, with time and the repetition of abusive episodes, the violence will escalate; the abuse will get worse. Emotional violence may be interwoven with physical violence to keep a woman trapped in an unacceptable situation: a negative and destructive cycle. This sort of situation of physical and emotional abuse has been compared with techniques used in prisoner of war camps to torture, brainwash and interrogate captives. This may include: 'Isolation, focus on the batterer's potential anger, exhaustion, dependency, feelings of incompetence, threats, occasional indulgences, degradation and humiliation, enforcement of trivial demands' (see Ginny NiCarthy, *Talking it Out: A Guide to Groups for Abused Women*, Seal Press, 1987, p. 100). If you are in a physically and/or emotionally abusive relationship you should seriously evaluate your options. Ask yourself honestly if your relationship is worth the price you pay for it – i.e. are the good times worth the bad? Does the 'cycle of violence or abuse' apply just to you or also to your children? Are you a victim of emotional abuse? If so, how? If you decide to change your situation, there are a number of resources available to you:
1. domestic violence counselling service
2. legal aid
3. women's refuges
4. Police Department
5. friends and family
6. solicitor
7. restraining order
8. Housing Commission
9. Social Security
10. independent finances
11. marriage guidance services (for you and your partner).

If you choose to stay in a relationship that is physically/emotionally abusive you'll need to think seriously about how you can make yourself safer and improve the quality of your life. And what about your partner? Can you get him to seek counselling and begin to attack the problem before it gets worse?

chapter 9

What to do if you are raped

Sweeping, though inconsistent, changes have been made during the 1970s and 1980s in Western countries' laws regarding rape. Rape is increasingly being addressed as a crime of violence and power, not lust; 'victim blaming' innuendo is under challenge; and more sensitive treatment of rape victims by those involved in rape cases has increased the number of women reporting rapes and the improved likelihood of convictions.

In the United States most States have adopted gender neutral statutes and redefined any sort of sexual penetration as sexual assault. Many have limited how much a victim's prior sexual history can be used as evidence in court; 29 States recognise rape in marriage as an offence. (See Louis Casamassa, *Rapist Beware*, Richmond Productions, USA, 1990, p. 44.)

To facilitate these legal changes and attitudes the definition of 'rape' has been widened into the term 'sexual assault' in all its varying degrees. This is the case currently in New South Wales. It is important to remember that laws vary considerably from place to place. For example, in England only actual sexual intercourse is recognised legally as rape.

The sexual assault laws in New South Wales, Australia, now state:

Sexual intercourse 61A. (1) For the purposes of this section and sections 61B, 61C, and 61D, 'sexual intercourse' means —

(a) sexual connection occasioned by the penetration of the vagina of any person or anus of any person by —

 (i) any part of the body of another person; or

(ii) an object manipulated by another person, except where the penetration is carried out for proper medical purposes;
(b) sexual connection occasioned by the introduction of any part of the penis of a person into the mouth of another person;
(c) cunnilingus; or
(d) the continuation of sexual intercourse as defined in paragraph (a), (b), (c). (See Sexual Assault Law Reforms in NSW, Dept of Attorney General and Justice, 1982, p. 8.)

The more violent the attack, the more severe the penalty. For instance, 'inflicting grievous bodily harm with the intent to have intercourse' has a maximum penalty of twenty years. 'Inflicting actual bodily harm' and 'threatening with a weapon with the intent to have sexual intercourse' has a penalty of twelve years.

Sexual intercourse without consent where the victim is over sixteen years has a penalty of eight years. Sexual intercourse without consent where the victim is under sixteen years has a penalty of ten years, but it is twelve years in cases where the offender is in a position of authority with regard to the minor.

Offences that fall short of sexual penetration but are classified as indecent assaults or acts of indecency carry penalties of between four and six years.

More recently (1988) there have been further changes in these laws to include:
- 'sexual intercourse procured by intimidation, coercion and other non-violent threats – penalty six years' (this means that if someone tells you that you must have sex with them or lose your job, they can be prosecuted under the sexual assault laws in New South Wales)
- 'sexual intercourse where the victim has an intellectual disability and the offender is in a position of authority – penalty ten years.

'Pack rape carries an additional two-year penalty on top of the basic offence charged.'

Also in New South Wales it is illegal for a husband to rape his wife. Also a woman's past sexual history is inadmissable in New South Wales. To a greater or lesser extent the changes in the laws regarding rape reflect a change in societal attitudes towards rape. The Kennedy-Smith trial in the United States, where one of the Kennedy clan was accused of raping a woman, received world-wide attention, as did the sexual harassment issue involving

Judge Thomas and Anita Hill. Though neither case lead to a conviction, they did focus much attention on the issue of sexual assault and gave notice to would-be harassers or rapists (even those in positions of power,) that not even wealth or position could any longer be guaranteed to immunise them from the legal process.

In a landmark interpretation of a 1984 jury verdict, Judge Barton of the Middlesex Superior Court in Massachusetts stated: 'No longer will society accept the fact that a woman, even if she may initially act in a seductive or compromising manner, has waived her right to say no at any future time' (Koss & Harvey, *The Rape Victim*, p. 132).

'No' means 'nothing further' and whatever past excuses may have been accepted on sexual arousal in males that could not be terminated, they are no longer tolerated by this society and by jurors who are a cross-section of this Commonwealth. Women are equal partners with men. They are not sex objects (Commonwealth v Crow, 1984).

What is your legal position if you defend yourself?

Usually half an hour into my classes someone will ask, 'What happens if in the course of defending myself, I kill them?' Then someone will ask, 'If I fight back, won't it make them more angry?'

Basically, this is an issue about fear. First, there is the perfectly understandable fear of arousing the attacker's deeper anger and provoking more violence by actively resisting or maybe even hurting him in the course of your own self-defence. Second, there is the natural fear of hurting, incapacitating, or, indeed, killing someone. Third, and not necessarily in this order, there is also the fear of confronting what lies within ourselves – the depth of power that most women haven't dared to use or even acknowledge. Women fear what might happen if they tap into these suppressed emotions that they have been sitting on for so long. There is the fear of what might happen if these emotions were allowed to surface 'in one hit'.

Let's deal with the question of what happens if, in the course of defending yourself, you wound or even kill your attacker. If you are genuinely defending yourself, then the attacker will have made the first physical assault. Basically, as soon as you are touched in an unwanted or abusive way, you are entitled legally to defend yourself with a justifiable amount of force. This means that if a man is harassing you and puts his arm around you, you must not shoot him (though you may feel like it), but you might bend his little finger if you have already given him a clear indication that his attentions are unwanted.

In some States of Australia (e.g. South Australia and Tasmania) the law actually allows the woman to defend herself if she has a reasonable belief that the man is going to attack her without him actually having had to lay hands on her yet. Speaking for myself, if I felt I needed to initiate an attack to survive I would rather be tried by twelve than buried by six.

The fear of making them more angry is the fear of death. Statistically it's the women who are more afraid of the rape who tend to fight back and the women who are more fearful of death who don't. Women who say to themselves 'I don't care what happens, this guy is not going to rape me' are the ones who fight back and statistically are the ones who get away, transforming their fear into a source of inspiration rather than immobilisation. There is an old saying: 'Courage is fear that has said its prayers'.

What to do if you are raped

The most important thing you need after you have been raped is support. Options:
1. Seek the help of a sympathetic and supportive friend.
2. Go to a rape crisis centre, a sexual assault centre, hospital, or community centre. Don't wash. You'll need to have the evidence.
3. You may ring the police or even go to the police station at this point if you wish to report the rape instantly. This doesn't mean you have to press charges and you can insist on a hospital examination/consultation with a counsellor before seeing them.
4. Get medical help — go to a hospital with a friend or counsellor. A social worker will see you at the hospital anyway. You must tell them that you have been sexually assaulted to receive the proper attention. The counsellor/social worker will present clear options to you so that you can make a decision as to whether you want to make a formal complaint to the police. Basically, the sooner you report the rape, the more likely it is that you will be believed.

The last thing you want is to go through this alone. The support you receive at this point will be a major factor in the degree of trauma the rape will play in your life. Without proper support you may feel like you are being raped continually, having to be examined and forced to relive the incident with no positive reinforcement. One woman who attended a workshop told me about being raped by two men in a country town. She said that the middle-aged male police officer handling the case kept reassuring her and saying 'No-one deserves to be raped', since she kept berating herself for being in the wrong place at the wrong time. This is the sort of understanding it is hoped rape victims will receive, but unfortunately it's not guaranteed.

The hospital

It is necessary for you to go to the hospital even if you are not physically abused and don't want to report the rape, because

- You may not know you are injured, or to what extent, as you may still be in shock.
- You may want to ease your mind about the chances of getting pregnant or of contracting a sexually transmitted disease. (Tests for these must be done in the weeks/months to come and cannot be done immediately, but you will have access to the morning-after contraceptive pill to greatly lessen your chances of pregnancy.)

If you decide to press charges or even just to give you the option to do so later, you can have the necessary forensic tests as well as a medical examination for injuries. It's important that you have these tests immediately because the longer you wait, the more chance there is that essential evidence will be destroyed.

If you are black, Asian, a lesbian, a woman from a non-English speaking background or a woman with a physical or intellectual disability, it is important that you get support from someone who is not going to be biased against you. You can request someone from your own background or support network as a counsellor and/or interpreter/advocate or at the very least someone who will go in and look after your interests. Be very aware that sexism isn't the only 'ism' you may confront at this point. This person can remain with you as your witness throughout the medical examinations, as well as when you make your statement to the police.

If you decide to make a formal complaint, you have a right to ask to be seen by a female police officer. You must go to the police station and make a sworn statement, which means you will have to go over what happened in detail and sign the statement at the end. The police will then investigate the case and if they decide that the case is worth pursuing they will arrest the accused and press charges. As a witness for the prosecution you will be required to attend a committal hearing where you will be grilled severely in cross-examination, more so than if the case goes to the District or Supreme Court — there are fewer constraints on the defence at this point. You will feel more like you are on trial than that you are a witness for the prosecution. This is because the defence (the accused's barrister) will somehow try and invalidate your statement by implying that you consented or that you were asking for it. In some States a woman's past sexual history is inadmissible, but remember that in this instance it's the defence's job to make you look bad. The accused (the rapist) is not required to give a sworn statement which means he doesn't have to subject himself to any cross-examination.

If the accused pleads guilty at the committal hearing, he will be sentenced in the District Court at a later date. If he pleads not guilty, the case will go to a District or Supreme Court for a trial by jury. If he pleads guilty he is free to change his mind any time before the final sentencing.

The jury must find him guilty beyond a reasonable doubt which means the jury must be really convinced he is guilty, no ifs, buts or maybes.

Compensation

You can claim compensation for expenses for your appearance in court. You can also file a civil suit suing the rapist for compensation, but he will not be charged by the police or sent to gaol. He will have to pay you compensation if you succeed.

You can apply for compensation for 'pain, suffering and loss of the enjoyment of life resulting from sexual assault, as well as for losses such as medical expenses and loss of income'. You can apply for this if no-one is caught, or even if the case is dismissed. The support organisation you use will give you information on how to do this. The amount of money you are entitled to claim varies greatly. In New South Wales it's $50,000 maximum.

What happens after

The response to being raped varies greatly from woman to woman. Many women rate it as the worst thing that has ever happened to them. During the process of reporting, going to the hospital, seeing a counsellor, you may even feel a bit numb, like in a dream, as if it's someone else doing it, not you. Many women experience this splitting off feeling in the course of, and directly after, being raped (the 'This can't be happening to me!' or 'I don't believe this!' feeling). Incest survivors also talk about experiencing this feeling.

Once you start to connect to your feelings again – thaw out from the emotional anaesthetic that shock produces – all sorts of other feelings may come rushing in. This will be effected by:

1. Your relationship to the offender. If it was someone close to you or someone you trusted, your whole world may be turned inside out because you then will ask yourself, 'If I can't trust him, then who can I trust?'.
2. The reaction of your family, friends and cultural background. In some cultures being raped is a stigma which means that you will be viewed as a ruined woman.
3. The treatment and support you received after the rape and the follow-up services provided. Obviously if the police, hospital, etc. were not supportive, then the emotional wounds will be much deeper.
4. The rape itself – the degree of violence, the length of it, when and where and how it happened.

The feelings you may experience include:

- feeling out of control of your life; loss of personal power. You may not feel brave enough to do what you used to do or to go where you used to go;
- fears and phobias (looking under the bed and in the wardrobe when you come home at night, checking locks and windows obsessively);
- shame and guilt: it's very hard not to feel as if you were responsible for what happened, that you in some way must have provoked the rape. Many victims, especially victims of date rape, blame themselves for just being 'plain stupid' – in this way they try to understand what provoked or led to a sexual attack. This is because women feel as if they are responsible for the sexual responses and arousal of men. Self-blaming is also a form of control and a way the mind will seek to gain control over a traumatic experience. For example, you may feel if I hadn't worn that dress then the rape wouldn't have happened, thus providing an explanation for the event, telling yourself

that if you never wear that dress again you won't risk rape ever again. Understanding the politics of rape is very important in order to allow you to move beyond this negative and unhelpful focus. The rape did not happen because of WHAT YOU DID, but WHAT HE DID.

Anger and indignation
These feelings are very healthy and natural. You have every right to feel angry at being abused. It is healthy to express anger, to let the pent-up energy escape rather than to keep it locked in.

Depression
Depression is anger that has been turned in on itself. You will feel this if you are not given an avenue or validation for your anger and indignation. If you are depressed, you need to communicate, express yourself and be given positive reinforcement.

Feeling cut off sexually
Sexuality is a vulnerable part of the human psyche. It's commonly the first thing to go when there is a problem in life. Obviously this is the part of you physically and emotionally that has been abused and it is not surprising if your sexual relations are affected for a while to a greater or lesser extent. Your sexual partner must be patient and understanding.

Flashbacks
The anxiety caused by the rape may lead you to have nightmares. Even when you are fully awake you may find yourself reliving the episode. A likely trigger for this flashback phenomenon is physical intimacy.

Phantom pains
You may experience this in parts of the body that have healed physically from the rape but retain the emotional memory of, that is, are associated with, the incident.

Reconnection with past abuse
Many women who are raped have been victims of sexual abuse previously, either as children or at other times. The rape then can have a much deeper or even a cumulative effect as it connects to other instances of abuse.

Feeling unclean
This is more likely directly after the rape. You may feel a strong need to keep washing yourself, to wash the violation away, to remove all traces of the rapist from you.

Fear that the attacker will return
This may not be unrealistic in some circumstances (e.g. rape in marriage), but most rapists are fearful of being caught and are unlikely to attack the same person twice.

Isolation
You may feel like nobody understands. Particularly if your family and friends act in well-meaning but inappropriate ways. For instance, they may be over-protective, not want to talk about it, blame you, blame themselves or think they know what's best for you. This is why it is often important to get added support from a counsellor trained in this area because they are not personally traumatised by what has happened to you, but can remain detached in a caring and constructive way. Ideally your support person will be a friend who is non-judgemental, understanding, and sensitive.

A self-help group, with or without a group leader, can be an extremely effective way of assisting the healing process, as it enables you to share experiences and work through the trauma. The attributes of such groups are directly opposite to the attributes of the forced sexual assault. In the same way that rape is the essence of an unsafe human relationship (i.e. it is violent, non-consensual and involves the abuse of power), the group provides a context in which closeness and intimacy can safely develop and finally thrive.

These groups may be long- or short-term, with or without a facilitator. You may simultaneously, or alternatively, choose to see a counsellor, therapist or psychiatrist, or you may find that you can work through the experience with the help of a few close friends – it all depends on the individual and the particular circumstances of the rape.

Exacerbation of addictive behaviour
If you are prone to substance addiction (alcohol, drugs, a food), a crisis of this nature may push you over the edge into real addiction and substance abuse in an attempt to blot out the emotional

pain. Support groups like Alcoholics Anonymous, Narcotics Anonymous, Overeaters Anonymous or Incest Survivors Anonymous are self-help organisations that can give you the extra support you need to deal with the addictive process.

A self-defence course

This can be a very valuable booster to your healing process. These classes provide an environment for the externalisation of anger and frustration through the punching and kicking, but without actually hurting anybody. They can stir the memory and the emotions, particularly as most self-defence courses include components in which discussion takes place and experiences are shared. Most women find the pure physical empowerment and the ability to do what they thought they couldn't (or shouldn't) are positive, empowering factors which help immensely to build their self-esteem and sense of control.

Other avenues

Other ways of dealing with the rape is to channel your anger into social or political action. Helping out at self-help groups is one alternative. Participating in marches such as Reclaim the Night can help you express practical anger (the personal is the political) for all women who have been raped. It hasn't just happened to you.

Collective self-defence

This is a case of a group from the community getting together and publicly confronting the rapist or wife-basher. It may take the form of several people talking to the rapist/basher in order to convince him of the error of his ways. (See Caignon & Groves, eds., *Her Wits About Her*, The Women's Press, London, 1984, p. 209, for examples of an American group called 'Women Against Rape' who employ this strategy.)

But this is not exclusively a Western phenomenon. In Maharashtra, India, when an Adivasi woman was raped by a landlord, the village women held a people's trial. The offender was publicly shamed. In another incident in Bombay, 500 people surrounded the house of a rapist and demanded that he be punished.

Some women in Germany and the United States have actively, after an extensive recovery program, confronted and counselled their rapists in gaol. Groups have been set up to change these men's attitudes and have apparently met with success, though it will take some time to say for certain.

To recover from a rape, a woman needs to make some sense of her experience and move on from it with confidence. Some victims discover inner strength they never realised they had, or a stronger empathy with others, in the aftermath of being raped. Some women decide to take action in their lives, and consciously leave the role of 'victim' behind.

The myths and the facts

MYTH Women enjoy being raped.
FACT No woman enjoys the violence and humiliation of rape. Sometimes women fantasise about being raped, but in fantasy the woman is in control. This does not mean she wants to be raped in reality.

MYTH A man cannot rape a woman if she doesn't want to be raped.
FACT Due to fear of death and physical violence, women may not put up much resistance because their fear makes them freeze. This doesn't mean that they want it, they just don't know how to stop it.

MYTH Some women ask for it because of the way they dress and act.
FACT The definition of rape is being taken sexually against your will, without your consent. What you were wearing at the time has nothing to do with you granting or withholding consent. No woman ever deserves to be or asks to be raped – no excuses, never ever.

MYTH Only young women get raped.
FACT Rapes can happen to anyone from babies to women in their 90s.

MYTH A woman can't be raped by her husband (she is his property).
FACT If you don't consent it is rape, whatever the rapist's relationship is to you – though the law lags behind in some States in affirming this view.

MYTH It won't happen to me.
FACT Rape can happen to anybody, including you.

MYTH   You can't defend yourself against a rapist – he is too strong.
FACT   You certainly can. Come along and find out how!

MYTH   Rapists come from a different class, race or culture to their victim.
FACT   Most rapes occur within a woman's own class, race or community (Bonney 1985). Certainly rape has also been used as a means to achieve racial and imperialistic domination, but for our purposes don't look too far afield for a potential attacker – you probably already know him. He more than likely fits somewhere into your normal everyday life.

MYTH   Rapists are strangers.
FACT   Over seventy per cent of rapists were known to their victims. (Bonney 1985).

MYTH   If you fight back, you are more likely to get hurt.
FACT   Fighting back does not determine the level of injury – if a rapist is going to hit you he will do it anyway. The more you resist, the more likely it is that you will get away (Bart & O'Brien 1985).

MYTH   Rapists are abnormal people, psychological monsters.
FACT   Psychologists have proven that the majority of rapists test normal – they are not dissimilar from most other men (Bart & O'Brien 1985).

MYTH   Rape is a crime that is motivated by an uncontrollable sexual desire.
FACT   Rape is a crime of power and violence that has to do primarily with domination and not libido.

MYTH   Rape happens in the streets late at night.
FACT   Most rapes happen in the victim's or the attacker's home or indoors.

(See Sydney Rape Crisis Centre, *Surviving Rape*, Redfern Legal Centre, 1990; Koss and Harvey, *The Rape Victim*; NSW Department of Health, *Adult Sexual Assault Information and Education Package*.)

Inventory for travellers
- Am I wearing clothes that enable me to use my arms and legs or run if someone attacks me?
- Have I got my awareness turned on when I walk outside the door, or is my head somewhere else?

- Do I walk confidently or like a victim?
- Do I carry something in my hands I could, if need be, use as a weapon?
- Have I checked my car to see if someone is in the back before I get in?
- Do I break up my walking, driving, parking routine so that my movements are less predictable to, and less able to be monitored by, a potential attacker?
- Do I allude to the fact that I am not alone, but have a large male companion who is due to arrive at any second, if I'm feeling unsure about someone?
- Do I stay close to the uniformed public servants when I am on public transport? When riding in taxis do I:
  1. Sit in the back?
  2. Book one ahead of time?
  3. Take note of the driver's details displayed?
  4. Make a complaint to his superior if he causes trouble?
- Do I hitchhike? Don't, it's too dangerous. He can take you anywhere and you will have no control. Get a bus, taxi, train or don't go.
- Are you assertive if someone is invading your personal space?
- Have I got tips from other travellers as to the best and safest places to stay (particularly from other women) interstate, overseas?
- Have I got all the necessary documentation in order — passports, visas, travel insurance, driver's licence (overseas)?
- Do I use a money belt or hidden compartment, not a handbag?
- Do I know the dress code and customs of the place I am going so as not to offend or invite unwelcome behaviour?
- Do I avoid taking any drinks, lollies, cigarettes or food — anything orally offered to you by friendly strangers when travelling, no matter how harmless they seem?
- Do I trust my instincts when I feel uneasy in a situation and remove myself?
- Do I always carry a map of where I am, and do I make an effort to never look lost?

(See also M. White, *Going Solo: A Guide for Women Travelling Alone*, STA Travel & Greenhouse Publications, Victoria, 1989; R. Baily, *Travelling Alone: A Guide for Working Women*, Optima, London, 1988.)

chapter 10

Psychological self-defence: *Prevention is better than cure*

So far this book has dealt primarily with the physical side of self-defence. Many attacks can be prevented if we practise our assertive skills, as well as our combative skills. These can be very important in preventing sexual or any other kind of assault since a very high proportion of attacks start off with a testing period to see if you are going to be an easy target. If you are assertive from the beginning it's likely you won't be targetted.

Let's consider, for instance, a situation which holds the potential for a date rape — most women will know exactly what I'm referring to. You have gone out to dinner with a man and allowed him to pay for your meal and at the end of the night he expects his money's worth. Now here we quickly get into an area that isn't either black or white. Where do we draw the line between the normal active/passive games men and women have been taught to play with each other (see 'Machismo' chapter), sexual harassment and actual sexual assault? How do we learn to communicate clearly what the limits are without our date thinking 'No' really means 'Just try a bit harder and eventually I'll succumb'? How do we clearly indicate that we are interested but don't want to have sex at this particular point in the relationship, or how do we get across directly and honestly that we are sexually interested and happy to take the initiative without being considered a nymphomaniac (which is the most polite label for what I imagine you might be called).

Despite the heavy pressure for women not to claim their sexuality, dare I say the more you are willing to acknowledge and tune in to your sexual feelings, the more you will be able to own them, make decisions about them and verbalise these decisions and feelings clearly to your partner. Some women just don't know what sexual attraction is. They are so used to gauging male sexual desire and doling out sex as a reward or a commodity that they remain out of touch with the intrinsic drive itself. I believe all men and women are sexual beings and it's a very basic function of our humanity to be so, as much for the survival of the species as for anything else!

When you are in touch with your feelings it's much easier to pull someone up when they stray over the line, because you are in touch with where the line is drawn as far as you are concerned. Thus many incest survivors have real problems in this area because the abuse they have suffered leaves them without a clear sense of boundaries. Being in touch with your feelings and accepting them as valid is crucial to your sense of self-worth and value as a woman, and contributes powerfully to your resolution and motivation to be assertive in your life.

In the two-day self-defence workshops I conduct the way the class strengthens their psychological self-defence is first to build up trust within the group. Members of the class are encouraged to share experiences, both successful and unsuccessful, of ways in which they dealt with assault or harassment. This is done first in pairs and then with the whole group. The strictest anonymity is stressed so that information shared in the group is not taken outside the group in a specific way. Also no woman is forced to disclose what she is not ready to disclose and women are also free to talk about the experience of someone they know in the third person if they prefer. These workshops are an important part of a healing and awareness process.

I then get the women to break into pairs to role-play a situation where one of the women must verbally de-escalate a situation using a strong voice, direct eye contact, powerful body language and the appropriate level of muscle. Part of the exercise includes naming clearly the behaviour they don't like and making use of external intervention.

Most of the situations we use in these role-plays are drawn directly from the participants' own experiences. They tend to fit into the broad categories of sexual harassment in the workplace, on public transport, in a pub, on the street, on a date, or with a friend/family member/spouse. Remember that harassment and assault exist on the same continuum – as a way of robbing women of their power and self-esteem. The quicker you nip it in the bud, the less chance it will grow into something uglier and more dangerous.

Once the women loosen up a bit and lose their self-consciousness about their acting ability they get right into it. They particularly seem to enjoy playing the harasser – don't ask me why.

Here is an example of a typical scenario we might role play; it is based on sexual harassment in the workplace – in this case an office.

Mr Jones (Anne's boss) comes and asks Anne to type a letter. As he speaks to her in a very flirtatious way he stares at her breasts continually. He then moves to the back of her chair and leans over her while explaining the letter to her as she is typing, all the time staring at her breasts. Anne says his name in a clear strong voice, looking directly at him and naming precisely the behaviour that she feels uncomfortable with or doesn't like, 'I would like you to look at my face when you are talking to me and not my breasts. Also I don't want you leaning over me when you are explaining what you want me to do as it makes me feel very uncomfortable'. In making 'I' statements and expressing her feelings about what Mr Jones is doing rather than what he is or by making accusations, calling him names or being abusive, Anne is attacking the behaviour, rather than the individual. She is setting her limits in an 'I am' way rather than a 'you are' way. Mr Jones then replies, 'Don't get paranoid, Anne, I was only being friendly'. She responds, 'Well, Mr Jones that may be, but I find it very invasive'. Here Anne is sticking to her guns and being persistent and clear.

We then discuss the role-play with the group and the consequences for Anne of being assertive. For instance, she may lose favour with her boss. We discuss ways around this, such as criticising the behaviour rather than the person. If necessary you can buffer the assertiveness by also emphasising some positive aspect of the person, like 'Mr Jones, I have worked for you for some time and found you generally a fair and reasonable person,

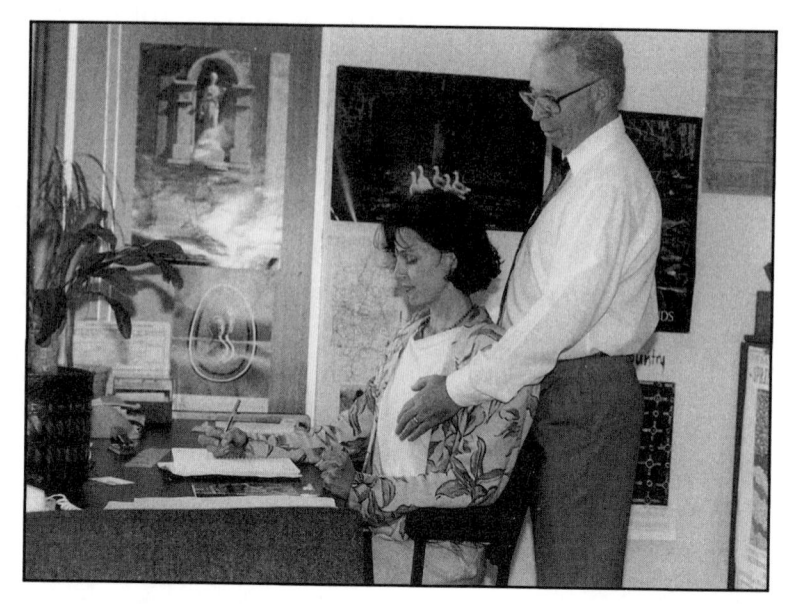

Safe in familiar surroundings at work? Sexual harrassment may come as an unwelcome surprise

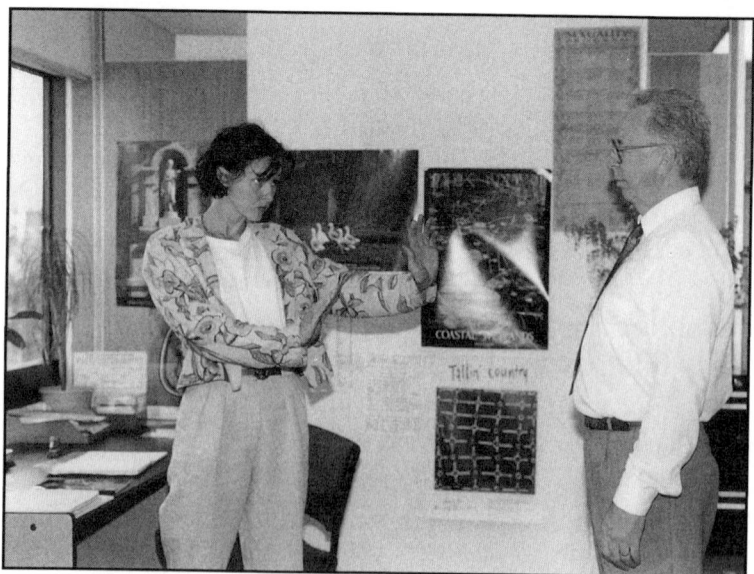

1. Use your voice,
2. eye contact,
3. defensive body language, and
4. create space between you and your harasser to get your message across: 'NO!'

but I don't like you staring at my breasts when you talk to me and I don't like you leaning over me, as it makes me feel uncomfortable. I value our working relationship and would appreciate you respecting my limits'.

We would then go on and discuss in the group the various options Anne would have and similar incidents that have happened to other women in the group or to people they have known. Options about taking further action if the harassment continues are also discussed. This may include writing the harasser a letter (factual and non-threatening), taking the complaint to the relevant sexual harassment officer, taking it to the Equal Opportunity Commission/Anti-Discrimination Board, taking it to the union. Anne could find out if other women in the office are also sexually harassed. They may offer support and band together to solve the problem.

However, this can't always be relied upon. For instance, one woman reported being continually harassed in the workplace by a senior male, but when she complained she was given the cold shoulder by the other women in the office because they believed she should have just put up with it, as they had learned to do. She felt that reporting the harassment had got her nowhere. On the other hand, a sexual harassment contact officer in a government department received a report that a particular man had approached a colleague when no one else was around and made a series of lurid suggestions. When confronted by the accusations, of course the offender denied them, though his misbehaviour continued. The contact officer advised the complainant informally to keep a tape recorder hidden on her person and to be ready to use it the next time this man made similar offensive suggestions. Strengthened with this evidence the contact officer was then able to properly confront the man and miraculously the behaviour stopped. (I don't believe this kind of resolution is in the sexual harassment manuals, but it proved effective in this situation. This informal strategy is by no means an alternative to correct procedure. You should consult your EEO officer as to the correct formal procedure and the policy of your department.)

Time magazine (21 October 1991) described a US example of successful sexual harassment litigation:

> Under Equal Employment Opportunity Commission guidelines issued in 1980 and unanimously affirmed by the US Supreme Court in 1988, sexual harassment includes not just physical but also verbal and environmental abuse. Under the law, there are two broadly recognised forms. The first involves a 'quid-pro-quo' in which a worker is compelled to trade sex for professional survival. In 1988 an Ohio woman won a $3.1 million verdict against an employer who invited her to perform oral sex or lose her job. (Nancy Gibbs, 'Office Crimes', *Time*, 21 October 1991, pp. 26-7.)

In New South Wales this form of sexual harassment is covered under the new sexual assault laws (sex through coercion) and faces a maximum penalty of six years' imprisonment.

Many women have found that simply reporting the behaviour has been enough to curtail it, only to find the harasser has changed his focus to the next new woman coming into the workplace.

Mostly the harassment seems to be between a senior male and a more junior female in an organisation. Many women have described how this can make it very difficult in terms of career advancement. Even though the law may be on your side it can take a lot of courage to confront the 'boys' club' that exists in many organisations.

But sexual harassment of course occurs outside of the workplace as well, such as on the way to and from work. One woman re-enacted being on a crowded train where she was being felt up from behind. She grabbed the man's hand holding it high in the air exclaiming, 'Who belongs to this?'. The man was glared at by the rest of the passengers and made a hasty exit at the next station.

Another woman related (to the great amusement of the group) the innovative way she'd found to talk her way out of being raped by a drunken yobbo who had dragged her into a shed. She had pretended that she was Norwegian and kept insisting that the man take her to 'a beautiful place' where they would 'make loove'. She kept saying in a thick Norwegian accent, 'This is not how vee do things in Norway'. The yobbo was swayed to take her somewhere else, en route to which she obviously made a quick exit.

After the re-enactment and discussion we move onto the use of body language as a preventative technique. The participants are asked to walk from one end of the room to the other in a victim's frame of mind. Then they are asked to give feedback on how they feel and how they are carrying their bodies. The usual feedback is that they take short steps with their eyes cast downward and are involved in their own thoughts rather than being aware of their environment. Their breathing is shallow and they move slowly.

The participants are then asked to walk assertively from one end of the room to the other. The feedback here is that their stride is longer, their head is upright and they are alert to what is going on around them. They walk quickly, take deep breaths and their arms move slightly as they walk.

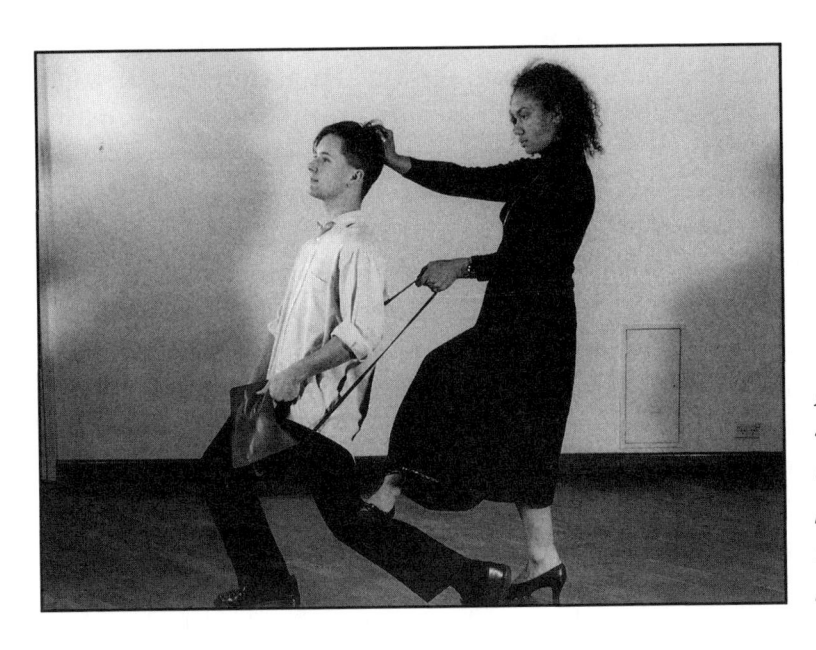

Bagsnatchers – the victim fights back! Grab his hair and heel kick down on the back of his knee as he flees

This exercise is very important because 90 per cent of communication is actually non-verbal. If you seem confident and strong you are less likely to be picked out for harassment or abuse. I had an experience of this coming out of a meeting in Kings Cross library, in an area infamous for drugs. A young man with pin-prick pupils (it was evening so this was a sure danger sign) asked me for money to get a taxi, as he claimed he was from out of town. When I refused and told him to go away, he commented how nice my bag was and how I'd better be careful or someone could snatch it. He said this as he backed away. My demeanour and tone of voice was enough for him to decide I was not the right person to pick for a bag snatch.

In the next part of the exercise the participants walk from one end of the room to the other in an exaggeration of empowerment swinging their arms, making lots of noise and taking up a lot of space (I call this my village idiots' convention exercise). This is lots of fun but can be pulled out of the hat for practical application i.e. no-one wants to attack a nut because they don't know what they are capable of doing. I have heard of women who find this strategy particularly effective when travelling late at night on New York subways.

It's important to reconcile the conscious memory with the subconscious motivation. This happens in the course of hypnotic creative visualisation (see exercises at the end of the chapter). I usually conclude the class or workshop with one of these exercises.

I also incorporate a bit of Swedish back massage as a reward for all the hard work done during the session. Sometimes I ask what did you like best about the self-defence workshop — inevitably someone will say, 'The massage'. I have found this technique very powerful in helping the information move beyond the head level onto a feeling level or, dare I say it, onto a spiritual level.

It's my belief that it's not skill reinforcement alone that will help women fight back and survive, but a gut-level decision and a shift in consciousness. This is why I prefer working with women initially in a two-day workshop format rather than in a week-to-week course, because this format gives more scope for the emotional shift to happen. The skill reinforcement can follow in the week-to-week classes.

I believe this emotional shift will enable the woman to match whatever situation she finds herself in with the tools available to her — be it a karate blow, a hammer fist, a loud voice, an assertive demeanour, a fast pair of legs, or a combination of the above.

The physical and emotional exercises work together and complement each other in heightening the effectiveness of the program.

Exercises

1. Make a confidential agreement with a partner and then share any experiences you have had in the area of sexual harassment or assault. Reverse roles.
2. Verbal assertiveness: with your partner act out these scenarios using the tools of a strong assertive voice, eye contact, body language, naming behaviour and increased level of muscle to deal with the harasser:

- being harassed in the workplace by a male colleague;
- being harassed on a train by another passenger;
- receiving unwanted advances from a man you have gone out to dinner with;
- being approached in a bar by a drunken stranger.

Reverse roles and give each other feedback.

3. Draw an anti-harassment network diagram — either work-related or another — so you can see the options open to you and the varying degrees of assertive 'muscle' needed, with information specifically relevant to your State or country.

Remember knowledge is power. The more options you are aware of the more power you have. It might be worth devoting a bit of time to researching your network.

4. *Anti-targetting exercise*
Working with a partner – one of you walk like a victim, and then walk assertively. The other partner observes and gives feedback on the body language. Reverse roles.
   Discuss feelings of being in each role – victim and observer.
   Discuss what you would look for if you were an attacker.

5. *Positive self-talk*
Stand in front of the mirror or in front of your partner and make five positive empowering affirmations about yourself. Your partner can give you feedback on whether your voice, eye contact and body language are reinforcing or cancelling your affirmations. For instance: 'I am powerful', 'I will fight back and succeed', 'I am a winner', 'I love myself enough to defend myself', 'I will learn to defend myself'. Reverse roles and give feedback.

6. *Office workers' exercise*
Notice at the next meeting in your workplace, who does most of the talking, who interrupts the most, who has the most power, who cancels whom, and how, after they have spoken. Notice the body language and personal space limits they have set. Notice who touches whom and how, and what sort of communication is happening. This may help you in your work as well as in your life.

7. Walk down the street making eye contact with all the men and women you pass. What sort of reactions do you get – sexual, aggressive, submissive, uncomfortable, indifferent, friendly, other?

8. How can you make dating safer? Discuss.

9. Which of your clothes restrict your movement and which enhance it? (I suggest that you measure your fashion purchases by this yardstick in the future.)

10. How can you expand your observation skills? Practise taking in everything that is happening in your environment. What can you see, hear, smell, taste and touch?

11. Imagine yourself as a man and write down what would be easier for you to do, what would be more difficult? Discuss.
   What wouldn't be expected of you, that would be of a woman? What would be expected of you, that wouldn't be expected of a woman?

12. *Empowerment guided visualisation*

Tape this visualisation, play it to yourself and/or your training partner in a comfortable meditative position with your eyes closed.

Close your eyes, breathing deeply in and out: breathing in positivity, breathing out negativity; breathing in strength, breathing out weakness; breathing in self-love, breathing out self-hate; breathing in courage, breathing out fear.

Picture yourself in a situation in which you are being attacked and visualise all the self-defence techniques you have learned. See yourself using them to fight off your attacker, committing them to your subconscious for when you need them, counting backward from 10: 10 - 9 - 8 - 7 - 6 - 5 - 4 - 3 - 2 - 1.

Feel your energy, feel your power, feel your self-esteem, feel your warrior spirit rising to give you strength to deal with any situation which you see in your mind's eye. Feel your power, feel your wisdom, feel your self-love motivating you to succeed, survive and thrive in any situation confronting you. Count upwards from 1: 1 - 2 - 3 - 4 - 5 - 6 - 7 - 8 - 9 - 10, and when you are ready you can open your eyes.

This is to be said slowly and clearly into the tape recorder and played at the end of each training session. You can embellish on this basic guided visualisation as you see fit.

These exercises can translate and transcend into other aspects of your life.

chapter 11

Women with special needs

This chapter examines the particular situations of women with special needs. Much of what is said can as easily apply to all women and so may be of more general use.

1. WOMEN WITH DISABILITIES

Women who have disabilities fight against the negative attitudes that have kept all women second-class citizens. Disabled women and children are the highest risk group for sexual assaults and abuse. With these things in mind it is obvious that people with disabilities should all be learning ways to protect themselves in order to improve their quality of life, bolster sagging self-esteem, and increase opportunities for dignified interactions and self-determination. (Kate Cloud and Judy Smith, 'Accessible Martial Arts Training is Good for Everyone', *National Women's Martial Arts Newsletter*, USA, p. 5.)

Women with disabilities have attended my regular classes, and I recently gave a class for a group of women with a broad range of disabilities. This class was small and required that I give each woman a large amount of individual attention. As for anyone beginning a course in self-defence, it is strongly suggested that you consult an instructor or medical practitioner before attempting anything too strenuous.

Women with disabilities have attended my 'regular' classes. The variables that determine how appropriate it is for a disabled women to attend a 'regular' class are:
- the attitude of the teacher
- the severity of the disability

- the size of the class
- the student's motivation
- the accessability and cost of the class.

Loss of a limb

If you have an artificial limb (prosthesis) you can use it as a striking and blocking weapon. The bionic woman of the TV series provides an excellent role model in this regard. If the limb affected is a leg, it may slow down your escape, also your balance may not be the best. Practice will improve these factors. Seek an external balance support, such as a wall or something sturdy to lean on.

Arthritis

This can range from mild inflammation of the smaller joints to total immobilisation of your whole body. I used to dread the arrival of an older arthritis sufferer in one of my classes. Her condition had turned her fingers into calcified stubs and her whole body seemed hard. Inevitably, I would get thumped and bruised by her hardened knuckles and joints, and she had no hesitation in hitting and hurting, believe me! Therapeutic Ayengar yoga classes are highly recommended for those who suffer from immobility, paralysis, tendonitis, strokes, blood pressure and scoliosis. Yoga is a gentle way to get the body going in preparation for something more strenuous. Arthritis is a temperamental disease that may change on a daily basis depending on the weather, diet and your mood; so work on days when it's happy and rest when it's angry.

Cerebral palsy

This may manifest itself in a lack of co-ordination, muscular weakness and damage to motor areas of the brain. Muscle tone can be overdeveloped and muscles may contract involuntarily. Accuracy may be a problem, as may co-ordination. This means that your mind can work faster than your body and you must allow for this delay. It also means that you must use the persistence momentum principle (hit often and hard, and get into what I call my I'm-in-a-bad-mood state), so that you may eventually hit your target. The erratic nature of your energy may be effective in itself as a deterrent to an attacker. Multiple sclerosis, muscular dystrophy, poliomyelitis, spina bifida can effect muscle tone, strength, movement and co-ordination, and in extreme circumstances your physical response may be limited. Generally speaking, the more localised the limitation, the easier it is to mobilise the stronger parts of the body. You may be in a position where you have to develop your verbal skills or look for resources outside your muscular body (e.g. alarms or weapons that require a minimum of energy expenditure – legal and licensed, of course).

Overweight women
Overweight women can suffer from a large range of physical problems, but the main barrier to them attending self-defence classes is psychological – the discomfort and fear of rejection caused by their poor self-image. Yet large women can come to love these classes, precisely because they can learn to use their weight functionally, in a positive way. Self-defence classes provide a fun way to get exercise and constructively 'throw your weight around'.

Anorexic women
These women can be severely underweight and may suffer from a similar self-consciousness about their body shape. Yet they need classes all the more since being small makes them more vulnerable targets, as does not feeling substantial in their dealings with the world. If they are serious sufferers from the condition, they may still perceive themselves as fat and incorporate the self-defence classes into a compulsive exercise program devised to burn off extra calories.

Depression and psychiatric disorders
The kind of emotional release self-defence classes give depression sufferers is enormous. This applies to a wide range of psychiatric disorders. The empowerment and uplifting of self-esteem may in itself open some doors.

Visual impairment
This can range from slight sight difficulties to total blindness. The blind are very sensitive to touch, so a blind woman will need a sighted partner to guide her body through the motions required for each exercise. The blind can develop a heightened sensitivity to sound, light and touch. The white cane can be used as a weapon of defence and the seeing-eye dog will discourage most attackers. If you are visually impaired to any degree, it is wise not to go where you are alone and cannot hear. If someone does grab you, quickly

assess where their vulnerable parts are likely to be from their position in relation to you.

Hearing impairment
Visual and touching cues are going to have more significance for a hearing impaired person. Any limitation of a sensory function may effect balance, co-ordination or muscular function.

Intellectual/developmental disabilities
Although more likely to be targetted for sexual abuse due to their vulnerability, these women have the same range of reactions as other women — from the very passive and lacking in confidence to the very angry and raring to go.

Women who use wheelchairs
Wheelchair use may arise for a whole range of reasons — degenerative disease, paraplegia, quadriplegia, amputation, broken bones and more. If the disability is restricted to below the waist, the upper body can be used for the purposes of self-defence. An inspiration to all those who are wheelchair-bound is Lydia Zydel who teaches self-defence and martial arts from her wheelchair. She teaches both disabled and able-bodied women.

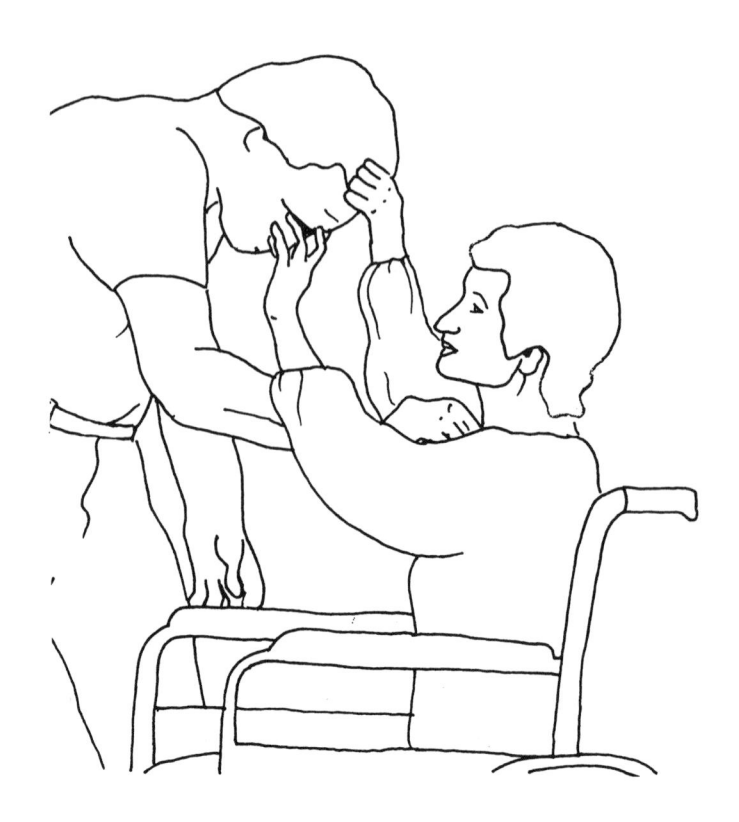

Disability inventory (for all women)

To help you evaluate your strengths and weaknesses and the ways in which you can improve your current abilities and attitudes, ask yourself:

1. Does your age effect how confident you feel?
2. How do you appear to the world? Do you have a disability that is obvious to other people? Are you heavy or light? Tall or short? Do you appear strong or weak?
3. How well do you hear? Could you hear someone walking behind you? Can you judge someone's distance or intention by the sound of their voice?
4. How well can you see? Are you long-sighted, short-sighted, totally blind, severely visually impaired? Do you take notice of what happens in your peripheral vision whilst looking straight ahead? Do you look people straight in the eye when you talk to them? How can you use your eyes as weapons?
5. Can you speak? Do you speak loudly or softly? Do you have a speech impediment that inhibits you in anger? Can you use your voice as a weapon?
6. Can you feel the sensation of touch on all parts of your body? Can you respond instantly to this, either positively or negatively? How can you improve on this?
7. How much mobility do you have? Are there parts of your body you can move and parts you can't? How flexible are you? Are you in pain when you move? Are you restricted in your upper or lower body? Do you have an artificial support you could use as a weapon?
8. How strong are you? Do you have strength in some parts of your body and not others? Can you maintain a position for a long period of time or do you need frequent periods of rest?
9. How fast are you? Can you change direction quickly? Do some parts of your body move faster than other parts? Does one part of your body slow down the rest?
10. How accurate are you? When you aim at something, how many times does it take you to hit it? How could you improve on this?
11. How fit are you? Can you sustain constant physical activity without getting exhausted? Can you exert rapid bursts of energy?
12. How long have you had your disability? Is it congenital or degenerative? Do you accept it? Was it the result of an accident?

Do you accept what you can and can't do? Is there room for improvement?

13. Go through this mental inventory: Are you in touch with the here and now, or do you live in a dream world? Do you believe that the world is basically a good place to be? Can you judge people's actions and reactions to you? Do you exude an air of confidence? Do you find it hard to say 'no'? Do you resent your disability? Do you feel the world owes you something? Have you ever been attacked? How did this effect your attitudes to other people and to yourself? Do you want to learn self-defence? Are you prepared to work hard for what you want? Are you committed enough to work hard for something, even if it takes a long time and may involve physical and mental pain?

14. Does your disability require you to have some kind of aid — cane, wheelchair, arm-rests of wheelchair that can be quickly dismantled, a prosthesis? Can these be utilised as weapons? (A weapon is simply a stronger extension of your body; what you can do with a fist or a foot you can usually do with a weapon.) Use this inventory to give yourself a thumbnail sketch of your strengths and weaknesses. If you have further questions related to your physical or mental health, you should consult a qualified professional before embarking on any dramatic change in your exercise, fitness or self-defence program. This section, deserves a book in itself. Apparently Lydia Zydel is writing a book on women with disabilities — a book to be awaited with much anticipation.

Note: The Disability Inventory has been adapted from Sandy Funk's 'Baseline Evaluation' Section II, in *Common Sense Self-Defence for the Aged and Disabled*, Pacific Press, Dallas, 1984, p. 7.

2. OLDER WOMEN: 'WEAKER IN BODY, STRONGER IN SPIRIT'

> 'I went to self-defence classes. In my mind I performed the exercises against this plunderer who strikes at vulnerable older women.'
> (A mugged woman's response as recorded in Louis Anike and Lyn Ariel, *Older Women Ready or Not*, Sydney, self-published, 1987, p. 86.)

Older women's attitudes to self-defence vary enormously, ranging from the 'If you try and take my money, I'll flatten you' to the lack of confidence that comes from extreme frailty.

On the whole, older women have a strength of spirit and a willingness to act which can compensate for a lack of physical strength. Lyn Ariel claims that some of this inner strength comes from the fact that since older women have sat longer on their anger, it is usually greater and a potential source of power. Also older women have not had the benefit of the range of services and heightened public awareness that is now taken for granted among the 'Baby Boomers', so older women have had to be more self-sufficient. It is easy to forget how tough and resourceful these women have had to be. That spirit is a great source of strength for older women to draw upon.

I prefer to teach older women in the context of mixed-age groups that involve children, teenagers, mothers and grandmothers. Almost without exception, these older women fight hardest, scream loudest, are the naughtiest (when I say 'Stop', they don't) and have a far better idea of translating what is being taught into action in a real situation. These older women are tougher, more determined and definitely more ruthless. They work around their disabilites and I suspect that age liberates them from all the Snow White expectations that hinder younger women.

In the course of a one- or two-day workshop, the younger women can usually maintain their energy levels, whereas the older women usually feel pooped by the end of the day, so in this sense they don't have as much stamina.

It is important to remember that chronological age is not necessarily the major factor in terms of being capable. There are, however, some general factors that do affect the aged population as a whole, and aged women in particular. Many older women are vulnerable to victimisation simply because they are alone, or depend on walking and public transport to get around.

Common physical problems are limited hearing and sight, arthritis, mobility problems, blood pressure, limited fitness and poor muscle tone. If you are an older woman with a disability you will probably need a class with a low teacher/student ratio, whether it be a general or a special interest class. In this way you should be able to get more individual attention and more easily progress at your own pace and achieve your maximum potential.

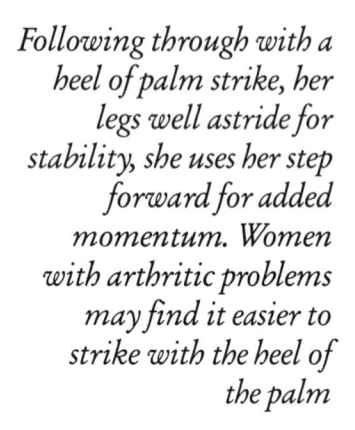

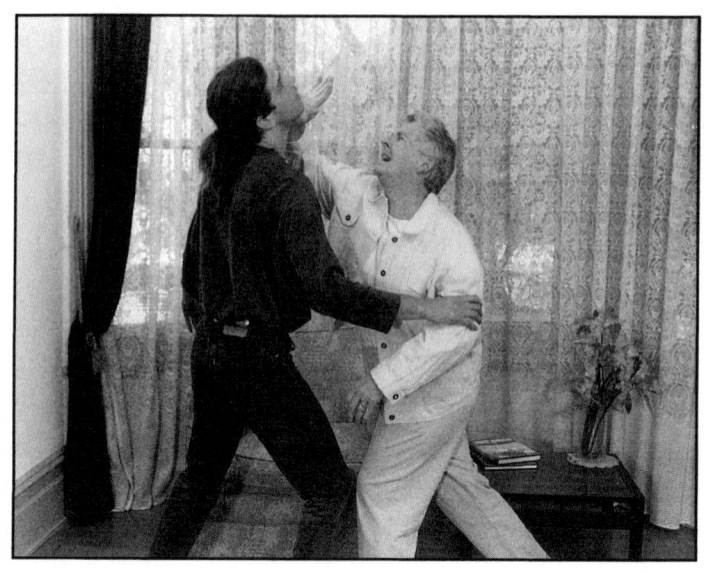

Following through with a heel of palm strike, her legs well astride for stability, she uses her step forward for added momentum. Women with arthritic problems may find it easier to strike with the heel of the palm

But remember, the only person you are competing with is yourself.

'It is much more likely that an older woman will be robbed rather than raped. The fear of being robbed or mugged is as much a limitation on older people's mobility as their actual "physical limitations and availability of transportation"'. (So reports Linda Lenoyer in her 'Harvey Survey 1974', *Self-Protection for Seniors – A Manual for Instructors – Alternatives to Fear*, self-published, Seattle, Washington, USA, 1981, p. 7.)

Purse-snatching and burglary are the most common crimes committed against the elderly. The 'granny' killings on Sydney's North Shore provided an exceptional circumstance where six fragile elderly women were murdered.

This doesn't mean that older women are not raped. There is probably an even higher incidence of under-reporting of rape for older women than there is for the rest of the community, given that most older women would feel shame that such a thing could happen to them. They were probably brought up with stronger taboos on discussing sex, much less discussing sexual assault. I would hazard a guess that sexual abuse may only be discovered if accompanied by some other form of brutal assault. Statistically, rape of older women accompanies other crimes.

When older women are raped, it nearly always happens in their own homes. A Philadelphia study revealed that 73 per cent of rapes of older women occurred at home, during a burglary (Linda Lenoyer).

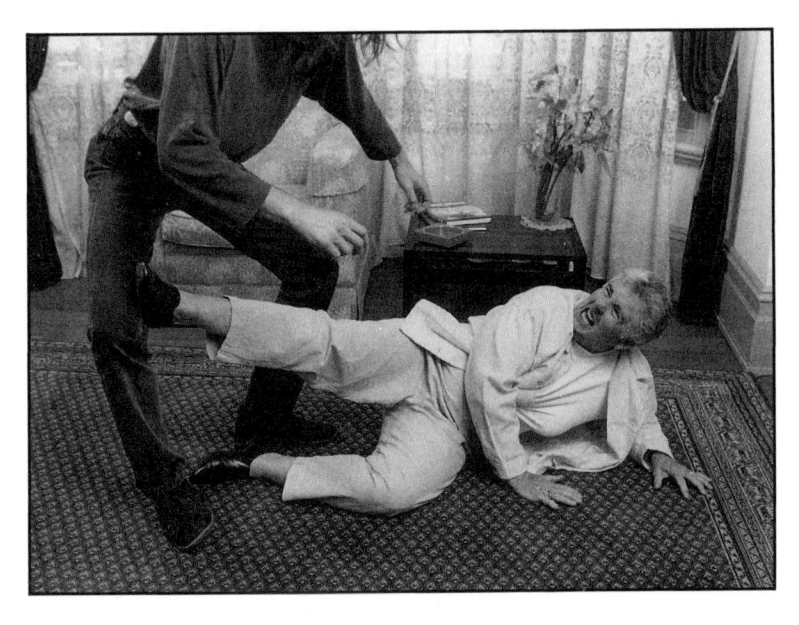

Good tactics. Bracing herself on the floor, she puts a well-aimed side kick to his vulnerable inner-knee, knocking him sideways. She will also be considering any available objects nearby that might serve as a weapon

Another source of abuse of elderly women can come from those well-known to the victim, and out of public view – physical or emotional abuse of a dependent older woman by family and caretakers. This could take the forms of emotional domination, physical assault, misappropriation of monies or the denial of adequate care.

This abuse may arise because of the inability of the caretaker to cope with the new vulnerability of a dependent relative, or it may be the by-product of a poorly run institution. (Lyn Ariel asks, 'Where are the refuges for older women?'). To avoid the possibility of abuse occurring older women should network as widely as possible with the community and not rely on any single family member or institution. In short, get an independent advocate to monitor your affairs – a family member, social worker, solicitor, friend, or member of a government department – particularly if you are severely incapacitated. The more vulnerable you are, the less isolated you need to be.

Household safety hints (for the young and the old)

(See also Sydney Rape Crisis Centre, *Surviving Rape* and the NSW Police Department's Community Relations Bureau's *Safety Advice for the Elderly: Some Simple Crime Prevention Tips.*)

1. Get a double-barrel deadlock.

2. Consult a locksmith about locks that are convenient, economical, provide safety and comfortable security (you don't want to feel like you're in prison).
3. Investigate the sorts of simple alarms and lighting systems that can be installed to make you safer, but not poorer (e.g. for the hearing-impaired a lighting system may be installed so that a light goes on when a window or door opens).
4. Install a peephole.
5. Never indicate to an unknown person that you are alone in the house.
6. Keep possessions out of view from, and out of reach of, windows and entrances.
7. Always have your key in your hand when returning home.
8. Don't let strangers inside your home without examining credentials. If you are unsure or suspicious, you can always ring the department or company concerned to check their identity.
9. If your place appears to have been entered in your absence, don't go into it by yourself.
10. Put security and 'Beware of the Dog' stickers on your door.
11. Create an agreed upon system of warning if there is trouble in your neighbourhood. Network strongly in your neighbourhood so that if someone intrudes there is someone close by who is prepared to intervene.
12. Assess your escape routes so you have a plan of action if someone does break in.
13. Avoid leaving doors open any time when unnecessary.
14. Don't go out without checking that the doors and windows are locked.
15. Leave the radio or television playing and a couple of lights on when you go out.
16. Check with Consumer Affairs if you are troubled by anyone trying to force you to buy or sell anything against your better judgement, or trying to get you to sign anything or to extract money from you for any purpose, especially on a door-to-door basis.
17. It is best to consult with a legal advisor or a trusted friend or family member before committing oneself financially to anything impulsively, particularly if it's someone who comes to your door.
18. Consult a security company about the cost of installing a security system — one that doesn't make you feel like you are in Fort Knox, but keeps you safe.

19. If it is convenient or pleasing to you, get a pet dog that barks loudly. If a dog is inconvenient, make a tape recording of a dog barking or a loud male voice that you can play when necessary.

20. Follow a schedule that's unpredictable.

21. If you come across a burglar, pretend you think he has a legitimate reason for being there (e.g. he is a plumber, gas man). This allows the intruder a non-confrontational 'out'.

22. Insert bolts into metal frames of sliding windows.

23. Take short screws out and insert long ones on all hinges.

24. Insert headless screws on outside hinges.

Safety tips when you are out and about

1. Whenever possible and convenient, avoid going out alone.

2. Walk in well-lit areas.

3. Be alert and aware of what's happening around you.

4. Learn to walk confidently and strongly in a non-victim-like manner.

5. Walk with large steps instead of small ones. Keep your head up.

6. Don't carry large amounts of money on you.

7. Be inventive in ways to carry valuables in places other than your handbag (e.g. sew large pockets into your coat to camouflage your valued possessions).

8. If you walk with a cane, carry it on the opposite side to the injured leg for better balance.

9. Before getting into your car, check the back seat.

10. Park in a well-lit area.

11. Don't put your name and address on a keyring.

12. Keep the doors of the car locked when driving.

13. Carry a personal alarm which can make a loud noise to attract the attention of onlookers.

14. Always communicate details of your comings and goings to someone close to you, so you are expected back at a certain time.

15. Have a good knowledge of public transport time-tables to avoid waiting around in isolated public places.

16. Keep a constant awareness of everything and everyone that makes up your immediate environment.

17. Sit next to a uniformed authority figure when travelling on public transport.

18. Develop a familiarity with using your possessions as weapons — torch, umbrella, hat pin, keys in between the fingers.
19. Your handbag may also be used as a shield to buffer blows from a fist, large instrument or a knife. You may want to use your handbag to block and your keys to strike.
20. Don't display money or valuables when you are out and about, and don't leave your handbag accessible and unguarded.
21. If someone is snatching your handbag it may be safer to let them have it and get a description of them than to actively resist.
22. You can tip out the valuables so they pick up the money only and leave your essential identification and keys.
23. Get money paid directly into your bank account and don't have cheques sent to you.
24. If you feel there are improvements that could be made in terms of transport, lighting or surveillance ring the appropriate council or government department or member of Parliament to let them know of your needs.
25. Contact the Police Department if you witness someone acting suspiciously in and around your vicinity or around other people's homes.
26. Carry a copy of this book to read on public transport.
27. If you are going away on holidays get someone to check your home or better still to stay in it.
28. If you're moving into a new home, install new locks (in case there are any keys in other people's possession).
29. Photograph valuables in colour in case you are robbed.
30. Don't discuss your valuables in public.
31. Dress for ease of movement.
32. If you are in care (a nursing home or with your family) get an advocate so that you have an independent monitor of your legal, financial and practical affairs. Don't be totally dependent on a single source of support.
33. Maintain a strong assertive communication with your care-givers. You should get and give feedback as to how things are going.
34. If you make a report to police or wish to warn people of suspicious types in your area, you will need to notice details — particularly anything distinctive or unusual. For example, try to remember their race, sex, height, weight, age, build, clothes, manner, voice, hair length/colour/or style, eye colour, and any facial or body scars or marks.

Exercises

1. Write a sentence on each of the safety tips and the relevance of each of them to your life and how you can implement them to improve your safety.
2. Write down three ways you can improve your safety by improving your networking in the community.
3. Make a constructive plan of action to help you overcome any fears.
4. Role-play with a partner that an intruder is coming into your house and then assess all your options (e.g. telephone, escape routes, shield, compliance, weapons, screaming).
5. Sit down and discuss how these options would change depending on the motivation and emotional state of the intruder.
6. One partner will walk like a victim and the other one will give feedback as to how this looks. Reverse roles. Now practise walking powerfully. Get your friend to describe the differences she sees in the two different ways you walk. Reverse roles. Sit down and exchange feedback on the different feelings that are triggered by the different walking styles.
7. Experiment with the best ways to hold a handbag. Get your partner to gently pull on the handbag and practise going with the pressure using a longer and lower stance. Practise getting it off your person if the pressure looks like it will make you fall. To do this in an extreme way you need a very padded surface and it should not be done in a lounge room – also work within safe limits. You should use this as an exercise to accommodate balance. You can:
   1. Practise falling (on a safe surface).
   2. Practise getting the handbag off your person so that you don't get dragged.
   3. Practise screaming to attract attention.
   4. Practise striking.
   5. Practise accommodating.
   6. Practise getting a description.
   7. Do a role play of someone pulling a confidence trick to gain entrance to your house, so that you can practise saying 'no' and being assertive using voice, body language and eye contact. Reverse roles.
8. Sit with your partner and talk about any disabilities you may have – your strengths and weaknesses. Assess the things you feel you could best do to defend yourself and the things you could do

least well and the ways you could compensate for this, if needed. Get feedback from your partner. Often others see more strength in us than we see in ourselves.

9. Brainstorm with your friend the ways to improve the general quality of your life. For example: What fitness classes are available and appropriate for your fitness level? Are there self-defence classes available? Are there yoga classes around that deal specifically with health problems you may have? Are there improvements you could make in your diet? Are there courses or community groups you would like to take or join? Are there community services you need that you have not yet had access to – home help, community nursing, Meals on Wheels? Are there ways you would like to contribute to your community by providing a voluntary service? Are there ways you could gain employment? Do you get regular medical check-ups? Are there alternative health measures you could investigate, such as acupuncture, herbal medicine, homeopathy?

10. Organise a meeting with your neighbours to figure out a safety code for your immediate neighbourhood.

11. Have emergency numbers displayed in a prominent place or memorise them.

12. Practise being grabbed and curling towards your attacker rather than letting your head pull away. You can tuck your head under your attacker's neck so you are harder to hit and harder to push to the ground. Do this gently at first with a partner.

3. YOUNGER (BUT WISER) WOMEN

I am particularly targeting women who are of high-school and university age, since so many of them come to my classes. I find that for this age-group it is important to stress the need for learning to nurture your new adulthood wisely, particularly to go through the material covered in the chapters on psychological self-defence and the machismo virus.

It is essential to be aware of dynamics which may confront you in dating situations at school or on campus. I especially stress the need to be careful in situations where drugs and alcohol are involved; all the more if you haven't had much experience with how these substances might affect you. (I know I sound like your mother, but maybe she is right. Remember that she was young once herself, she wasn't born a mother.)

Above all, this is the age when you are searching for and formulating your adult identity and it's very important to be true to yourself:

> The problems start when the partners aren't fully mature: when a woman isn't confident enough to express herself and when a man isn't sensitive enough to care about what the woman, is feeling. In the heat of passion men don't always hear what's being said, and women – especially those who are naive, inexperienced and uncomfortable talking about sex – don't always express themselves quite as forcefully as they should. That's why date rape is prevalent amongst teenagers. ('Date Rape', *Cosmopolitan*, Australian Consolidated Press, April 1993, p. 124.)

4. WOMEN OF COLOUR, ASIAN WOMEN, AND WOMEN FROM NON-ENGLISH-SPEAKING BACKGROUNDS

Racism is a powerful force that can often put women in a more vulnerable position because of their 'differences'. You should seek out a non-racist instructor who will empathise with your experience. Pick someone for example with whom you feel comfortable and who will cater to any special need you may have. Alternatively, you might be able to choose an instructor from your own background who will better understand your situation.

5. LESBIANS

If you are a lesbian looking for a class be careful as to whom you 'come out to'. You probably will feel more at home in an all-woman, pro-feminist, pro-lesbian environment:

> A survey of 252 lesbians at the 1991 Lesbian Conference in Sydney revealed that:
> 72% of women had experienced verbal harassment, 40% physical intimidation, 15% physical violence, 10% sexual assault, 13% domestic violence, and 28% had experienced no harassment. All these statistics were from the past twelve months (Statistics from *Lesbians on the Loose*, Issue 28. Vol. 3, no. 4, April 1992).

6. THE CHILD WITHIN (INCEST SURVIVORS)

Many women who have been survivors of child sexual assault and incest often have only got in touch with the memory of this experience in their adult lives. Often it is advisable to seek the support of a group or qualified counsellor to work through the emotions that have been locked up inside.

Victims of sexual abuse will often shut down emotionally because this is how they coped when the abuse occurred. This makes feelings hard to recognise or name. Moving in a self-defence workshop may help some women to connect with these denied feelings and help the mind and body to connect with the inner life.

I believe that we store emotions in various parts of our bodies or at least associate different significant events with specific parts of the body. In the course of doing self-defence, the movement of bodily parts in an assertive and deliberate way may provoke these deep emotions. Anger is a common emotion that is released or experienced in these sessions. Punching, screaming, and yelling can provide a healthy release for stored legitimate anger. The self-defence class can help to translate this emotion into positive, self-affirming energy. Remember, if we don't find an escape hatch for our repressed emotions we cannot begin to heal.

Some women have gathered the courage, strength, commitment and inspiration from the self-defence workshops to then go and confront their abuser.

chapter 12

The martial arts: *Which one?*

Women's self-defence instruction has two frames of reference: one is feminist, one is not. My approach to both martial arts and self-defence starts with the premise of empowering women. The other, more martial-arts based approach, springs from the notion that women can take on a more 'male' energy when they strike back. This latter approach focuses on 'stranger danger', that is, that women just need to respond to events; it doesn't confront societal values regarding power between the sexes. It therefore pays to consider *which* martial art and *which* teacher is right for you.

Make no mistake, I recommend you do a short-term women's self-defence course before deciding to take up a martial art. Even if you have been studying martial arts for some years, I suggest you do a short-term self-defence course anyway, because you will develop a very practical context in which to apply martial arts principles. Also, if the martial arts style you've been trained in primarily functions from a front-on, standing position, you would be well advised to take a self-defence course, since it is most likely that you will be approached or attacked from behind and end up having to defend yourself from the ground.

The criticism I tend to get from the martial arts community is that you can't possibly learn enough in the short amount of time available for a typical self-defence workshop — for example, over an intensive weekend. My answer is that you can learn plenty, but hopefully you won't stop your training there.

Women will ask me if six hours are enough, are twelve hours enough, are twenty-four hours enough training? I would

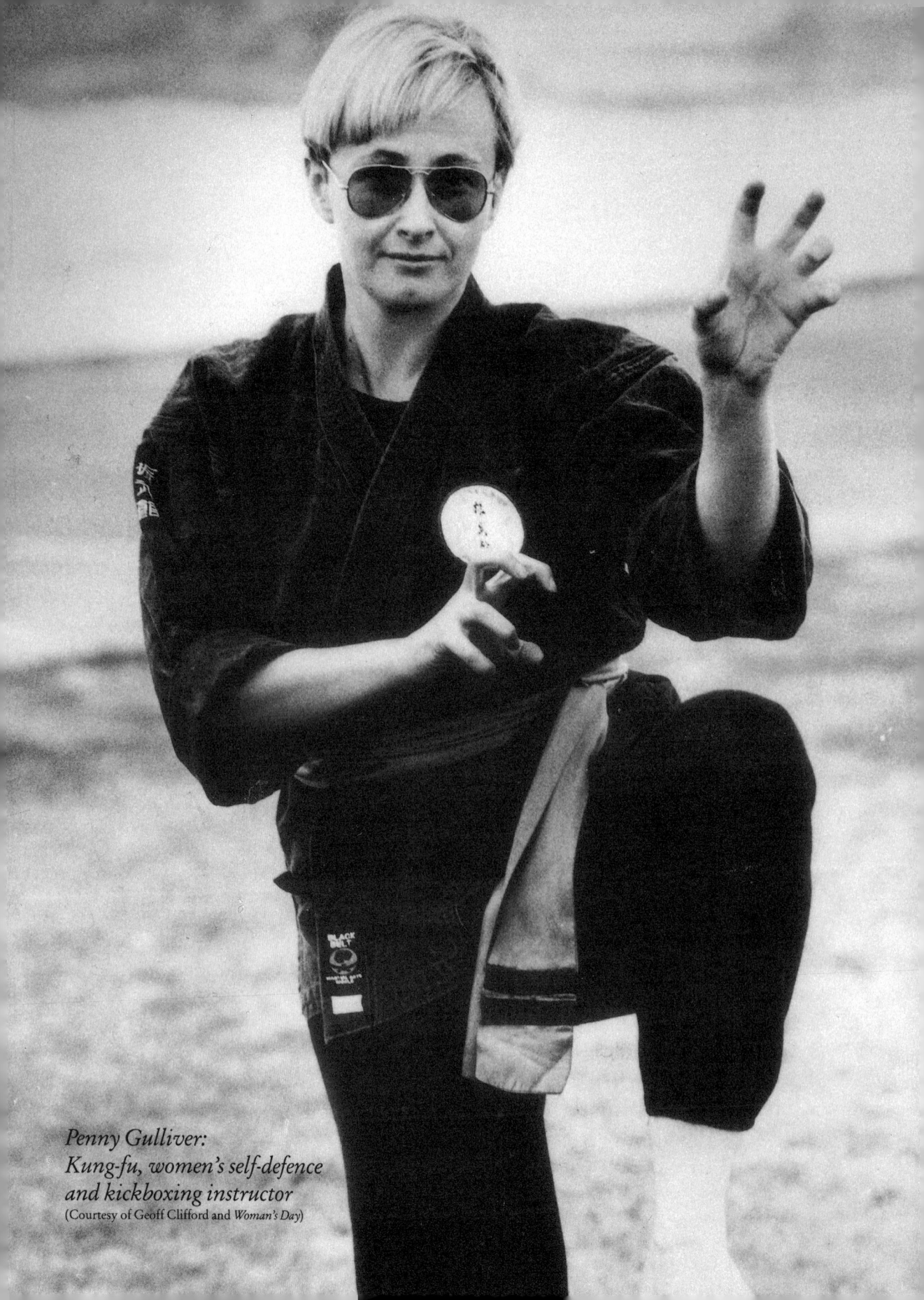

Penny Gulliver:
Kung-fu, women's self-defence and kickboxing instructor
(Courtesy of Geoff Clifford and *Woman's Day*)

suggest that ideally you continue some form of training (either self-defence or martial art) for the rest of your life, three times a week. (It is recommended that for your general overall health and fitness you engage in some form of regular exercise three times weekly — so why not make it a self-defence or martial arts class?) The least I would suggest is an annual refresher, if you have already got the basics from a course. Failing that, do it yourself in your own time at home. Get a video (such as my *Self-Defence for Women*, Seven Dimensions, 1990) or use this book to practise with regularly at home. Obviously the more you practise, the better your skills will become.

Having taken a self-defence course, which of the martial arts best suits you? If you decide not to train in a martial art, then you can always go on to take an intensive advanced self-defence course.

Martial arts is for people who want a long-distance run, not just a short sprint.

Initially I studied women's self-defence in 1975 under Maggie Brooke at the Rape Crisis Centre in Sydney. I have since studied a number of styles, and teach Kung Fu and kickboxing. The style I have primarily studied since 1977 is called Jin Wu Koon with Sifu Chan Cheuk Fai. I chose this style because it combined the harder straight-line principles of karate with the soft circular movements of Kung Fu. (I have now created my own style called Women's Kung Fu.) The style had a strong weapons component as well. I found that I could get both traditional and fighting skills in the one place and the training atmosphere was supportive and inspiring. So you see it it is very important to find a club that suits your needs.

To assist you, here are some questions and answers relating to the style of particular martial arts and the teaching and atmosphere of the different clubs. To my mind every style is good and can be given practical applications, but some are easier and quicker to apply than others. What follows is a simple thumbnail sketch of the various martial arts you might like to consider:
- Are you looking for a style which teaches you immediate fighting skills and where the goal is to learn to hit, kick, knee, elbow hard and often — is quick to learn and involves little obvious traditional training? If so, *Muay Thai* or *kickboxing* is for you. The classes will consist of kicking, hitting, elbowing, kneeing, punching bags either held by a partner or hanging

from a wall, sparring (pretend fighting with protective equipment), fitness work (skipping, sit-ups, push-ups — most styles include this component). Muay Thai actually has a soft rhythmical flow which is surprising, considering its devastating effect. The Muay Thai classes I have attended provided a lot of one-to-one training with the instructor holding and wearing the bags and the students laying into them. (I have found it far more fun being instructed than being the instructor in this context!) You can train to fight in full contact competition or you can train just for fun with low-key or even no sparring (in any style you should be able to choose the level of intensity of your sparring).

- Are you interested in a style that has a strong traditional structure, is linear, with an element of self-defence training? *Karate* is a good place to start if you're seriously thinking of taking up a martial art over a long period of time. It stresses stances, discipline and Budo — spirit development. Many clubs still retain close connections with their roots in Japan and Okinawa.

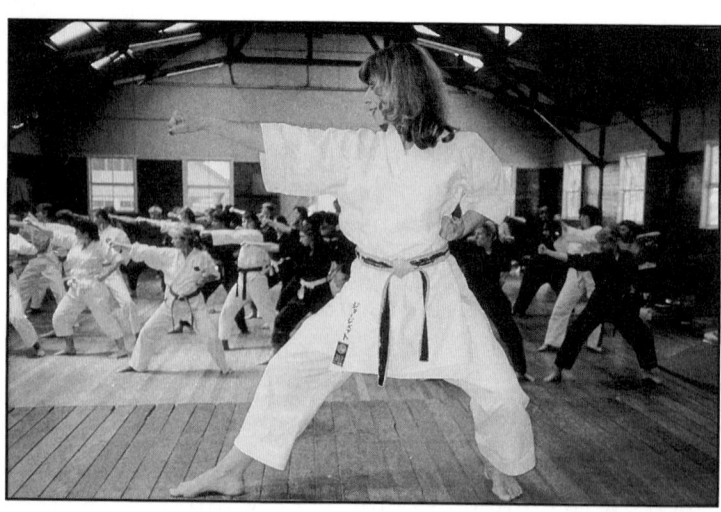

Georgette Dyett presenting Shotokan karate at the Kata workshop, Australian Women's Martial Arts Federation Camp, Sydney

Others prefer to do their own thing and improvise a bit. Karate is definitely a style that will earth you and give you some grounding, but with a sharp rhythm if this is what you need. You also get awarded belts — as grades from white through to the universally recognised black, as a symbol of martial arts achievement (though black belt means you are only ready to start high school, not graduate).

Karate schools vary enormously in their orientation. I call karate a 'hard' martial art because it relies a lot on the muscular

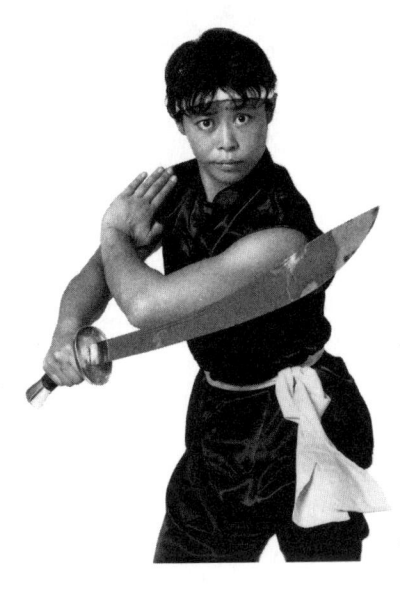

Janet Gee, a Choy Lee Fut exponent in San Francisco, demonstrates the use of a Butterfly knife. This is a traditional Kung-fu weapon; although it is usually very blunt and has not been used for fighting in this century
(Photograph courtesy of Terry Lee)

contraction at the point of impact and rapid retraction of a punch or kick. Techniques of karate may include breaking boards, punching, kicking, blocking and kata (forms). You get to wear a white uniform called a gi. Some clubs participate in sport karate (semi-contact), pulling the punches up one inch from the face, but hitting the body hard in sparring.

Different clubs emphasise different things. Here are a few examples. *Shotokan karate* is a style that is traditional with low stances and a very linear technique. *Kyokushin-kai* is a karate style that has hard training and full contact sparring techniques – a tough style. *Goju* is a mixture of the hard, straight-line technique and the softer, more round technique (softer doesn't mean you hit softer or that you are weaker – you actually hit harder through softness). *Wado-Ryu* is a more circular defensive karate more influenced by the Chinese arts.

- Are you looking for a more circular 'softer' art which you can use for self-defence and which bears a relationship to animal forms? *Kung Fu* is such a martial art. Just as all roads once led to Rome, so all roads lead to Chinese Kung Fu when you are looking for the origin of the martial arts. In all martial arts there is a lot of overlap.

There are many types of Chinese Kung Fu. Most combine an external component to improve the strength, speed and stamina with an internal component connecting you with your Chi energy or life force. This doesn't rely on your external strength, but more

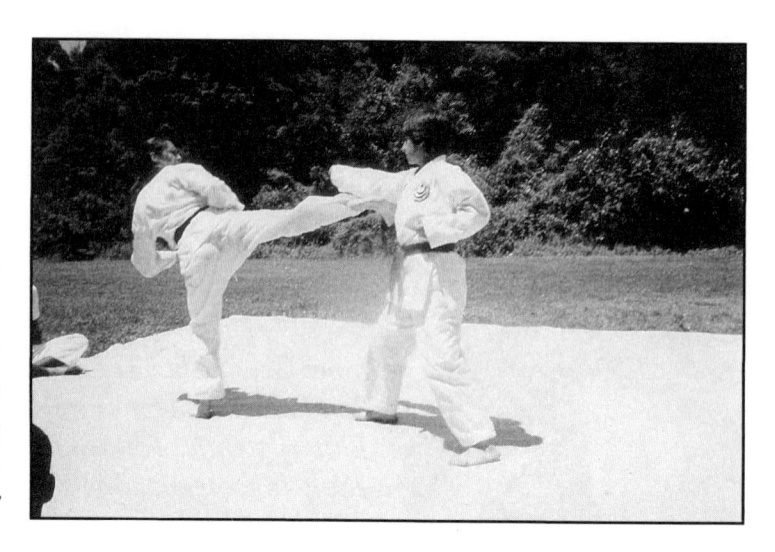

Tae Kwon-Do

Carol Middleton demonstrating Tae Kwon Do kicking techniques in Washington DC

on your 'connection' with your opponent and with your ability to channel the energy being directed out towards you back to your opponent either 'nicely' or 'not so nicely' – depending on what is thrown at you initially. So the energy goes full circle. (All of the arts stress spiritual significance, sometimes obviously, sometimes subtly.)

Here is a description of a few popular Kung Fu styles: *Wing Chun* – a style primarily using hands with short deflective movements and simultaneous punching and blocking with a vertical fist. Invented by a group of Shaolin monks, including a Buddhist nun called Ng Mui, Wing Chun prides itself on having a practical application which can be achieved in a short space of time. Wing Chun will suit a shorter person acting in a close-range situation.

Praying Mantis – a circular style that imitates the movements of this insect.

White Crane – this style combines the long, sweeping movements of the crane, with a high stance.

Choy Lee Fut – employs strong, wide, sweeping movements, stances are low. Provides weapons training. The hard and soft components imitate animals, such as the monkey, snake, tiger, crane and dragon.

Wu Shu – this is a very gymnastic style flourishing in China. It has lost much of its fighting application and is now basically a mixture of Kung Fu form, ballet and gymnastics (great to watch and good exercise).

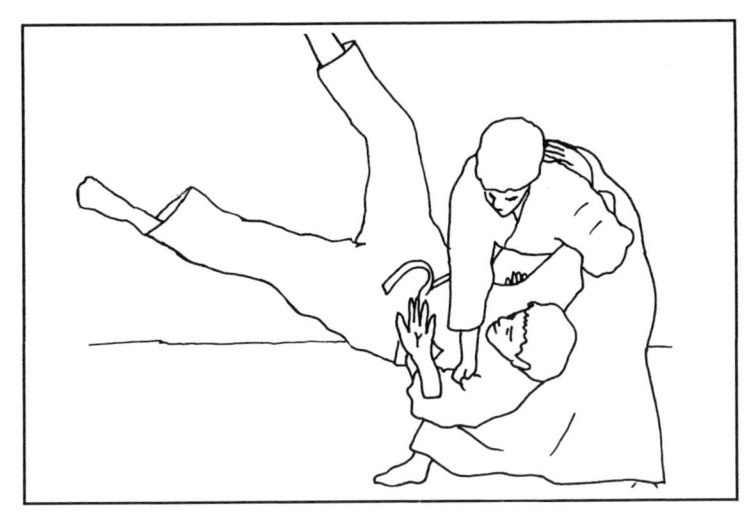

Jujitsu

Jin Wu Koon — is a mixture of Northern and Southern styles characterised by long stances. It also has a strong karate influence.

- Are you looking for a style which primarily improves your health and is spiritually enriching and is less immediately concerned with teaching self-defence? *Tai Chi* looks like Kung Fu in slow motion (take it from me, it's a lot more strenuous than it looks). The main principles are relaxation, balance, slowness, consistency with a never-ending, flowing quality. Tai Chi is connected strongly with Taoism. I would not recommend Tai Chi for those wanting to get quick streetwise answers, but if you learn the more martial applications of this art, the effects can be devastating.

- Are you after a style which has a lot of high fancy and sometimes flying kicks, as well as hand and self-defence applications (70% kicks, 30% hands)? *Tae Kwon Do* is a Korean-based art that features lots of kicking — of advantage to women in that anatomically the legs and hips are where women have a lot of power. Clubs compete in tournaments and there is no shortage of places to train. There is probably a centre somewhere near you.

- Are you interested in a style that teaches you to fall, throw or apply locks? Any style where you learn ground techniques is very important and can improve your self-defence knowledge. *Ju Jitsu* is the mother art for these arts. It is the most directly self-defence-oriented of these falling and throwing arts, incorporating strikes with locks, throws and falls, often with bone-breaking applications (but not when practising).

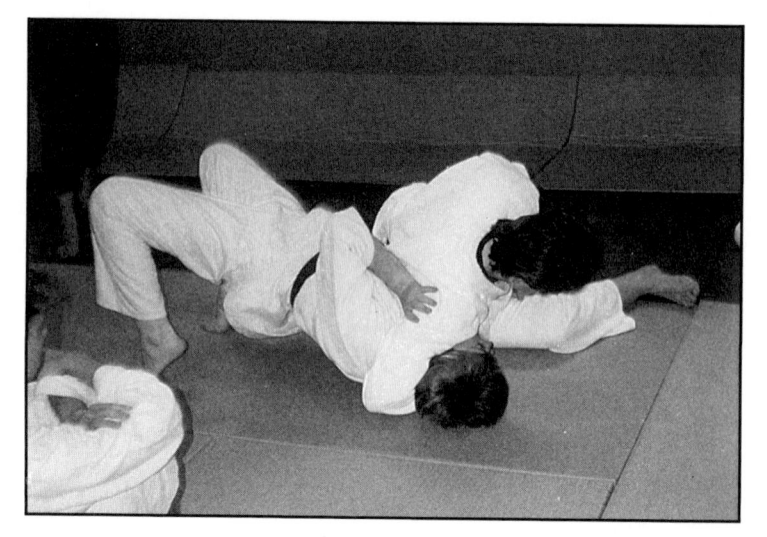

Judo workshop demonstrating ground techniques, Women's Martial Arts Camp in the Netherlands

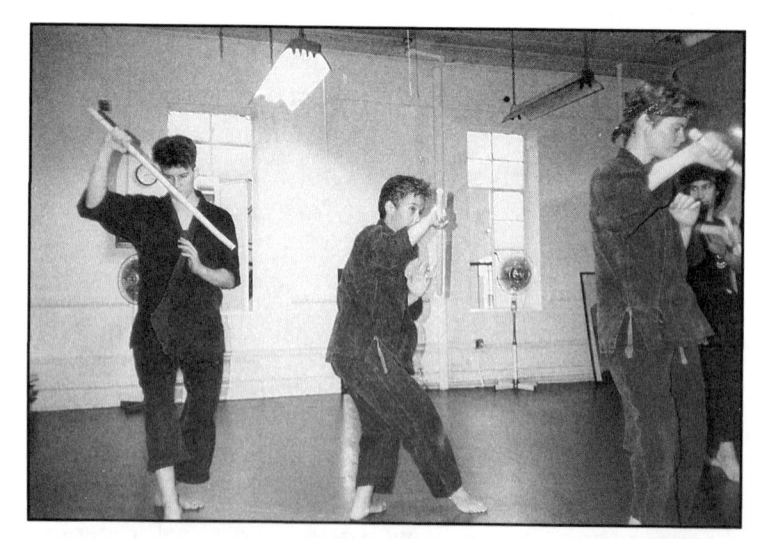

Annie Elman and students practising Arnis, or Philippino stick fighting, Brooklyn Women's Martial Arts, New York

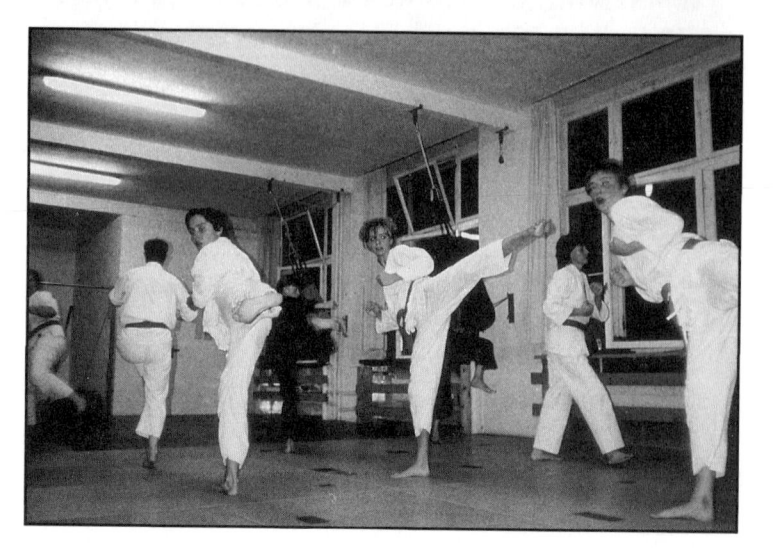

Wado-Ryu karate class in Berlin (world's largest women's dojo)

Judo is not a martial art as such, but a sport derived from a martial art — a bit like Ju Jitsu, with the strikes and nasty bits (the bits you need to know) taken out. Good for learning falling and throwing. Judo is an Olympic sport and provides a lot of opportunity for women to compete.

Aikido meaning 'the way of harmony' is another Ju Jitsu derivative with a lot more 'do' ('way') than Ju Jitsu. Aikido is a non-violent way of directing negative energy from your opponent away from you using locks, throws and falling without causing harm to your opponent. This martial art is steeped in the philosophy of balance and harmony and is not appropriate for those seeking a quick solution, but it is good for the soul.

- Are you interested in an art which is gymnastic, acrobatic, done to music and which will allow you to do a handstand or cartwheel as you kick your opponent in the head? *Capoeira* is a Brazilian style invented by the black slaves working the cane fields. It's acrobatic, dance-like and comes in at you at unexpected angles. A style that's appropriate for the more agile.

- Are you interested in a martial art that will give you a little bit of everything? There are several of these.

    Hapkido is the one that comes to mind. This is a Korean-based art which has high kicks, throwing and falling, leaping often in the air and falling (not in your first lesson), locks, self-defence, breaking techniques. It's not sport-orientated, but self-defence-oriented — a good smorgasbord style.

    Tang Soo Do is another Korean-based style giving a mixture of kicks, locks, falls and throws with some opportunity for competition. This style has a strong spiritual philosophy.

    Ninjitsu has a long history of self-defence effectiveness as it was developed by medieval Japanese secret agents and assassins. (Today real ninja are more likely to wear business suits and carry guns.) Again there are many aspects to this art: throwing, falling, camouflage. A good all-round style.

- Do you want an art that will teach you about weapons? Most of the arts just described have a weapons component. Usually you learn unarmed basics and then you are introduced to the weapons' component of the art using the same combative principles you learned in hand-to-hand combat. The weapon

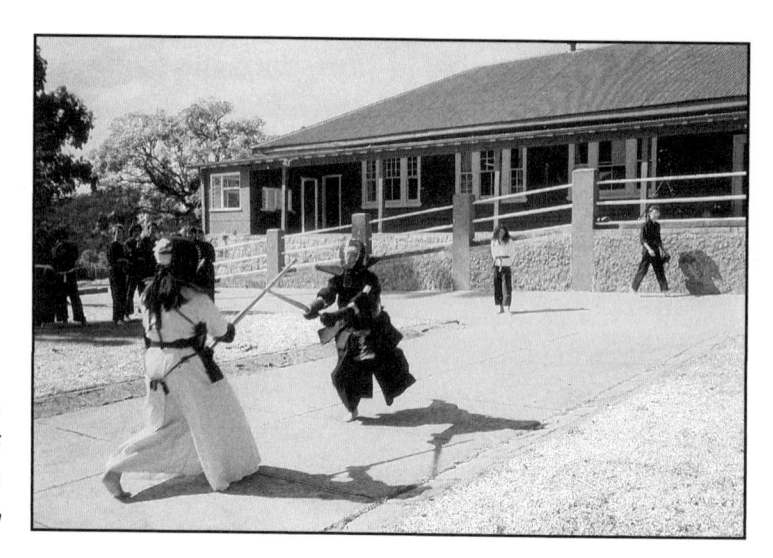

Kendo demonstration, Australian Women's Martial Arts Federation Camp, Sydney

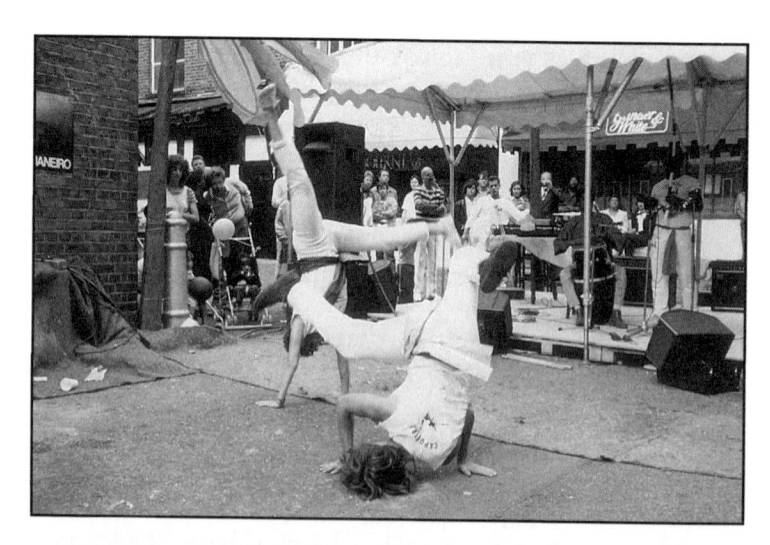

Capoeira exhibition in London

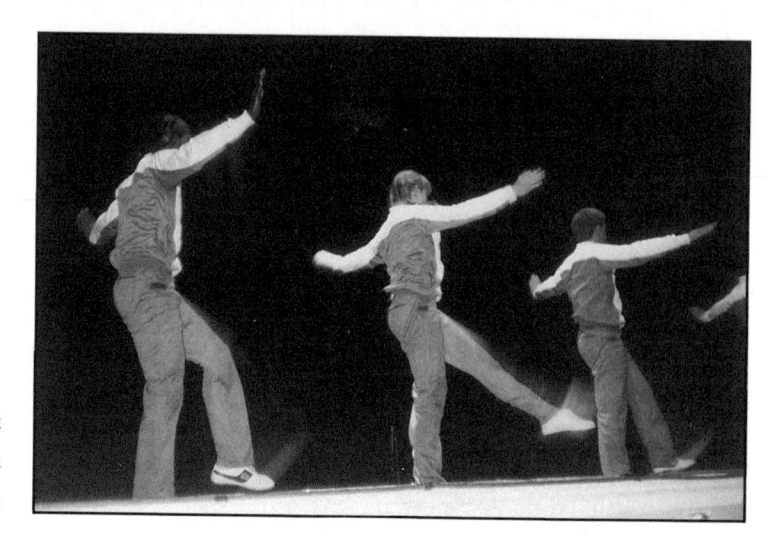

Wu-Shu demonstration by the English team in London

then becomes an extension of your hand. This could be a sword, a long stick, a chain, sai or two short sticks joined together with a chain. (I have been tempted to invent a modern-day woman's weapon out of a pair of high-heeled shoes taken off the feet and worn on the hands — excellent weapons with their pointy steel tips.)

Kali Arnis, Escrima, is the exception — if you want to get straight into weapons. A Filipino art which emphasises the use of twelve-inch long wooden sticks as well as knives and other weapons. Kali has a very effective anti-weapons component. (A lot of weapons are actually made from very simple implements. Peasants, banned from possessing conventional weapons, were forced to use their ingenuity and cunning and fashion weapons out of the everyday objects available to them. This is something to bear in mind when you find yourself unarmed and in need of a weapon.)

Arnis is an extremely pragmatic style based on direct street experience. There are now Arnis competitions which involve heavily padded competitors, striking one another.

- Are you looking for a weapons-based martial art which is purely an art form and is not so concerned with actual, practical self-defence? *Kendo* is a traditional art derived from a very deadly one. Protected by a lot of padding and armour and a large bamboo stick, your object is to hit your opponent on the head, wrist or mid-section. Most Kendo practitioners make no pretence about the self-defence aspect and participate purely for the love of the art.

- Are you interested in a style that moves from high to low stances and has an unpredictable and unusual rhythm? *Silat* is an Indonesian style that has only surfaced fairly recently because it was kept secret and not shown to many Westerners — an unusual style because a lot of it is applied close to the ground.

- Are you interested in learning about a weapon that has been traditionally designated to women in Japan? In more war-like times, Japanese women used a long stick tipped with a blade, the *naginata*, to protect themselves at home while their husbands were away. Nowadays the blade is replaced by wood, and opponents are heavily armoured. Unless you are in Japan, you will be hard pressed to find a class offering instruction in the use of this weapon. Nevertheless, it's worth mentioning this art because of its status as a women-only martial art.

- Are you interested in a style that primarily uses pressure points? Now this is a very controversial topic in martial arts circles. Most of the arts I have mentioned have a pressure-point application system. These points in the hands of an expert can apparently be used to knock out or even kill an opponent. Whilst many in the martial arts community remain sceptical, I keep an open mind on the subject, having been knocked out and revived by pressure-point applications. This knowledge can have profound ramifications in teaching self-defence, but it is not appropriate for the purposes of a short-term course because of the intricacy and exactness required.

The styles I have mentioned are but a handful of what is available. There are many breakaways and mixtures of styles on the market, but often it's not what style you are taught, but how it is taught. You can make any style work for you if you want it to.

Just because you have learned a martial art doesn't guarantee your safety. For instance, I once received a call from a martial arts instructor about two women he had trained to black-belt standard. They had just returned from a two-month intensive training program in Japan. The problem was that the lower grade males were going out of their way to be extra rough with these women and the women would react by dissolving into tears. This instructor wanted to send his black belt women to me so I could teach them how to fight!

Now obviously if you are learning an art with a larger, stronger person (irrespective of sex) and your ability level is roughly the same as the larger, stronger person's then they can beat you. Usually, when you have to defend yourself, you will find that your attacker has ensured that you are in the position of the weaker, disadvantaged party, and so you are left with few options but that of having to fight 'dirty'. My advice to these two women would be to: (1) make sure you can choose your practice partners – get permission from your instructor; (2) confront these men verbally when they get out of control, don't tolerate abuse; (3) accidently on purpose slip in a few very painful below the belt strikes and apologise profusely afterwards (works for me); (4) persevere – use your instincts as to how you can best deal with the situation; or (5) leave this club and come and train with women where you will rarely encounter a meat-head.

I have encountered this situation many times myself and avoiding these idiots is the best way. It's best to network with the higher grades because they are usually (though not always) more secure within themselves and have less to prove.

If you are forced to teach or compete with men who feel they have to test you out, you must pass the test. Show you are strong and tough on their terms because unfortunately meatheads only understand the language of pain.

Do you want a place where you can dabble in a wide variety of martial arts so you can choose the one that suits you best and do so in a safe and supportive atmosphere?

The Australian Women's Martial Arts Federation runs annual camps, dedicated to the unity and betterment of women in self-defence and the martial arts. Any women is free to go and try out a whole variety of martial arts in a friendly and supportive environment. I personally spearheaded the formation of this organisation after visiting the National Women's Martial Arts Federation at the USA training camp at Yale University in New Haven in 1986. I also visited a similar camp in the Netherlands shortly after. The women's martial arts movement has been functioning in the USA since 1972, so we have been able to learn a lot from our North American and European counterparts.

Here are some questions you may want to ask to decide whether or not a particular club is right for you:
1. How many women train in the club?
2. How many women are in senior grades in the club?
3. Does the club have a woman instructor/instructors?
4. Does the club have only women instructors?
5. Does the club have only women students?
6. Is the style one that interests you and one that you would feel comfortable doing (you will feel a little inadequate at first no matter what style it is because it is new, so don't mistake lack of confidence with lack of initial ability).
7. If there are men in this club what feeling are you getting from them:
    (a) Is the instructor fair to female students?
    (b) Are there meatheads in the classes who would make you feel uncomfortable and threatened?

(c) Do the women seem to get less serious attention in class than the men?
8. Does the class go at a pace you can manage?
9. Does the class 'feel' right for you — are you getting good vibes? Does it look safe — are there many accidents?
10. Is it convenient?
11. Is it in the right price range?
12. Realistically, how often are you going to get there?
13. Are you prepared for a short-term commitment or a long-term commitment?
14. What is the standard of the beginners?
15. What is the standard of the seniors?

Most clubs will give you a free lesson. It is best to take advantage of this and try several before you buy.

Where do I go?

The Australian Women's Self-Defence Academy will teach anywhere in Australia (the world, for that matter) on a workshop basis, or week to week. If you want information about self-defence classes, martial arts courses, or the Australian Women's Martial Arts Federation in your local area, direct your inquiries to:

PO Box 266
Bondi Beach
NSW 2026 Australia
Ph: (02) 308 064   Fax: (02) 365 6253

If you are looking for a locally based course, we will recommend one in your area, or else you should contact your local Department of Sport and Recreation, Rape Crisis Centre or YWCA, or your local Sexual Assault Centre or Women's Information Centre. All of these centres usually run courses or will be able to refer you to courses or martial arts near you.

For information about self-defence in the USA and UK, contact:

Carol Middleton
701 Richmond Avenue
Avenue
Silver Spring
Maryland
USA 20910
Ph: (301) 589 1349

National Women's Martial Arts Federation
Melanie Fine, Treasurer
PO Box 4688
Corpus Christi
Texas
USA TX
Ph: (784) 69-4688

The Martial Arts Commission
Broadway House
15-16 Deptford Broadway
London SE8 4PA
Ph: (01) 691 3433

Appendix

Warming up

This chapter will merely skim the surface of a very important subject that extends far beyond defending yourself. The important thing is to approach your exercise routines creatively, always remaining conscious of safety and of setting yourself clear, manageable goals that you work towards in a gradual and realistic manner.

All exercise requires a degree of warming up and, as a rule of thumb, the more vigorous and gymnastic the exercise, the more warming up is needed. In addition, each individual needs to assess their own limitations. If you have a physical injury or disability, you must work within your limitations. On the other hand, you also need to extend your limits safely, gradually, and sensibly. I mean you don't go and run a marathon if all you have done for years is walk to the corner shop to buy milk, puffing if the shop is at the peak of a slight incline. (Before I embarked on a course of self-defence and martial arts, my own exercise routine consisted of walking from the television to the refrigerator. This was twenty years ago. I now train a minimum of three times a week for between one-and-a-half and two-and-a-half hours, despite a heavy work-load.)

Meeting regularly with a training partner can encourage you both to practise and make it easier to use equipment. It's usually preferable, initially, to practise with someone who is at an equivalent level, and of a similar weight, size, and strength, since most women tend to get discouraged if they are outclassed too much, too soon.

To warm up, do five to ten minutes of either jogging or jogging on the spot, skipping, aerobic dancing, exercise-bike riding, jumping around. Whatever you do, do it fairly moderately, just enough to get the body moving and the circulation flowing.

To cool down, do five to ten minutes of stretching at the end of the workout: this is when the body is most receptive to stretching because it's warm and it's necessary to unwind the tension.

Stretching exercises will help maximise your range of movement. Stretching also encourages blood flow through the joints and increases the elasticity of the muscles and ligaments. Stretching should always be co-ordinated with the breath, so that you are exhaling as you reach for your maximum point of extension, inhaling as you relax the stretch. To improve your stretch, you should hold each position for at least thirty seconds. If you are only doing a quick warm up, you should hold each position for about ten seconds. Stretching should be relaxed and a relaxing activity. Your breath should be even, rhythmic and deep, allowing the energy to flow through the joints.

How you breathe is very important to how you feel, to your emotions and to your ability to externalise your power. Try a stretching exercise while holding your breath and then try it co-ordinating your breath with the movement and notice the difference. You may try the same experiment with one of the punching exercises.

A bit of brute strength never goes astray if you are fighting off a six-foot Neanderthal. You could incorporate half-body push-ups graduating to full-body, abdominal exercises or the routine use of light weights. This can be included in the warm-up section or at the end of your self-defence routine.

Push-ups

Go down onto your knees for push-ups. If you're doing the full-body version, which you can do if you've got a fair bit of strength in your arms, make sure not to curve the lower back. Your bottom has to be straight or slightly pointing up, so that you're not doing push-ups with a sway back. It's no good having a concave spine, because if you do, you risk injuring your lower back. If you can't do full-body push-ups properly or you find them unduly strenuous, it's better to do half-body push-ups (that is, from the knees), and gradually build up strength. The main thing when you're doing push-ups is to keep your elbows in; however if you are doing push-ups specifically to develop your triceps, then perform the push-up with the biceps and elbows out. Standardly your feet are together, your elbows are in, your bottom is slightly up and your back is not concave. As you push up, breathe in; and as you come down, breathe out.

Most women would be advised to start off doing push-ups from the knees and build up strength. But when you do them from the knees, make sure the knees are well back so that you're not cheating.

When you get really good you can do push-ups one hand on top of the other, or you can do them on your knuckles. But usually it's best to do them on a soft surface. (Children are ill-advised to do push-ups on their knuckles, since their bones are still growing.)

Other variations are to do push-ups with the hands next to each other, with the hands under the shoulders, and with the hands wide apart. If you are doing half-body push-ups, remember that in order to build up your strength you must constantly push yourself beyond your previous maximum capacity. So, for example, if you start off doing ten, then you can increase the number of push-ups at your own pace, until perhaps you are doing not ten, but sets of ten.

Abdominal exercises

For your upper abdominals lie on the mat to do a sit-up. Bend your legs so that your heels are touching your buttocks, your hands are clasped on the side of your head, your elbows are wide and you slowly round your spine and putting the emphasis on your abdominal muscles, so that you're tightening your abdominal muscles as you come up slowly, touching your elbows as much as possible to your knees, rounding and crunching your abdominal muscles, and then slowly going down. Breathe out as you come up, and in as you go down. Repeat ten times.

Then for lower abdominals you're going to lie flat with your hands under your head and you're going to bring your heels to your buttocks. Straighten your legs to the perpendicular, but with your knees slightly bent so that the pressure doesn't go into your lower back. You're going to slowly lower your legs to the ground. Then as the heels touch the ground, bend your legs in towards your buttocks, then straighten them up again and then slowly lower them to the ground. So your legs go down to the ground, your heels touch the ground slightly, your knees bend and then they come back up to the perpendicular. You're going to bend your legs again. (This is for your oblique muscles and for your waist). Still lying down, you're going to bend your knees and touch your elbow to the opposite knee, hold it for one second and then come back down again and repeat ten times, holding each time for one second.

Each of these abdominal exercises should be done slowly with concentration so that the stomach muscles are being utilised rather than putting any strain on the lower back. If done quickly with weak abdominals, there is a tendency to refer the stress to other areas of the body, usually to the lower back. Don't forget to exhale with the exertion.

An exercise for strengthening the lower back is to lie face down on the ground, put your hands under your hips palm up and slowly raise both legs off the ground, keeping your chin down and then lower your legs, focusing on using your lower back muscles. Do this ten times.

If any of these exercises cause any pain that goes beyond the pain of exertion, stop immediately, do it more moderately or substitute an exercise with which you feel safe and comfortable.

Remember: When in doubt, leave it out.

Running away from an attacker is your most effective self-defence tool. If you practice running and sprinting regularly you can improve your speed and endurance. So every woman should do some form of exercise to improve her stamina and speed. Jogging with sprints of say 50 metres would be ideal for incorporating speed and stamina. This is best done separately from your self-defence routine, because it is too tiring to do both consecutively, unless you are very fit.

Your workout then consists of 15 to 20 minutes of warm-up (stretching), 20 to 60 minutes of cardio-vascular activity and 10 minutes of cooling down (stretching), plus a few minutes of meditation and so on.

Generally speaking, to improve your aerobic fitness you have to do any activity that uses the large muscular groups that can be maintained continuously in a rhythmic and aerobic fashion, such as, in running, jogging, walking, hiking, swimming, skating, bicycle-riding, rowing, rope skipping, and various endurance games and activities. The activity will ideally be maintained for 15 to 60 minutes, will occur three to five times per week and will be done at 40 per cent to 60 per cent of one's maximum heart rate. This level of activity will enable you to reap the benefits of aerobic activity: a lower resting heart-rate, a bigger heart chamber with thicker walls, a more efficient level of working muscle, and a lower risk of developing heart disease.

Training with a martial arts class is an ideal way of doing your exercising, because at the same time as you are strengthening, flexing, and gaining all-round aerobic and anaerobic fitness, you are also learning to defend yourself. Generally speaking, you'll find that you will get more all-round fitness and exercise from a martial arts class than from a self-defence class where the emphasis is on defence strategies and self-protection rather than on fitness.

Bear in mind that it takes a lot of energy to fight back when you are attacked, and, if you're not very fit, then the amount of energy you have over and above your emotional energy will quite likely be in short supply. Obviously the fitter you are, the more you can do to defend yourself and ward off an attacker.

> **Warning:** Before beginning a fitness program of any kind it's advisable to consult a medical practitioner and a qualified fitness instructor and/or martial arts instructor to establish a suitable program.

If you want to find out more information pertaining to designing a fitness program, there are some excellent books referred to in the bibliography. Alternatively you can go to your local gym and have a fitness assessment designed by a qualified instructor adding your self-defence moves to this. Health and safety are your number one priority. Don't overdo it – remember the tortoise got there first.

Bibliography

Adult Sexual Assault Information and Education Package, NSW Department of Health Sexual Assault Education Unit, February 1990.

Anderson Bob, *Stretching*, Shelter Publications, California, 1988.

Anike and Ariel, *Older Women Ready or Not*, Anike/Ariel, Sydney, 1987.

Anti-Discrimination Board Annual Report 1990-91, Sydney.

Anti-Discrimination Board Guidelines for Employers – Eliminating Sexual Harassment, ADB, Sydney, 1987.

Atkinson, Linda, *Women in the Martial Arts*, Dodd, Mead & Co, New York, 1983.

Baily, Roberta, *Travelling Alone: A Guide for Working Women*, Optima Press, London, 1988.

Balaskas and Stirk, *Soft Exercise*, Unwin London, 1983.

Bart and O'Brien, *Stopping Rape: Successful Survival Strategies*, Oxford, Pergamon, 1985.

Bass, Ellen and Davis, Laura, *The Courage to Heal*, Harper & Row, New York, 1988.

——, *The Courage to Heal Workbook*, Harper & Row, New York, 1990.

Brownmiller, Susan, *Against Our Will: Men, Women and Rape*, Penguin, London, 1976.

Butler, Pamela E., *Self-Assertion for Women*, Harper & Row, San Francisco, 1981.

Caignon and Groves, eds, *Her Wits About Her*, The Women's Press, London, 1984.

Casamassa, L., *Rapist Beware*, Richmond Publications, USA, 1990.

Connell, R. W., *Gender and Power*, Allen & Unwin, Sydney, 1987.

Curry, Lisa, *Total Health and Fitness*, Angus & Robertson, 1990.

D'Arcy, Tony, *Workbook Sexual Harassment Contact Officers Workshop*, Canberra, Harris Van Meegan Consultants Pty Ltd, 1991.

Fighting Women News, vol. 12, no. 2, Summer 1987.

Funk, Sandy, *Common Sense Self-Defence for the Aged and Disabled*, Pacific Press, Dallas, 1984.

Gibbs, Nancy, 'Office Crimes', *Time Magazine*, 21 October 1991, pp. 26-7.

Holland, Jones and Stewart, *Self-Defence for Women – Woman to Woman*, Golden Press, 1987.

Iyengar, B. K. S., *Light on Yoga*, Allen & Unwin, London, 1984.

Koss and Harvey, *The Rape Victim*, Sage Library of Social Research, 1991.

The Law Reform Commission of Victoria Report, *The Unsworn Statement in Criminal Trials*, September 1985, (Minority report presented by J. A. Scutt), p. 28.

Leung, Debbie, *Self-Defense: The Womanly Art of Self-Care, Intuition and Choice*, Washington, R & M Press, 1991.

Lewis, Peter, *The Way to the Martial Arts*, Golden Press, Australia and New Zealand, 1990.

London Rape Crisis Centre, *Sexual Violence – The Reality of Women*, Womens Press Handbook, London, 1984.

Lucas, Jan, 'Sexual Harassment: Current Models of Occupational Health and Safety and Women,' *Australian Feminist Studies*, Autumn 1991.

Mioche, Anne-Marie, 'Martial Arts – A Different Sport', *Active-Women in Sport Newsletter*, Summer 1992, pp. 12-13.

Morgan, Jenny, *Sexual Harassment, One Man's View, the Einfeld Decision*, Refractory Girl, Sydney, 1989.

Nedea, A. and Thompson, K., *Against Rape*, Farrar, Straus & Giroux, New York, 1974.

Nelson, Joan M., *Self-Defence: Steps to Success*, Leisure Press, 1991.

Ni Carthy, G., *Talking it Out: A Guide to Groups for Abused Women*, Seal Press, 1987.

NSW Sexual Assault Committee Report 1985-1987-1988.

Peddy, Lisa, *The Heathen, Heretics and Holy Women of the Feminist Pedagogy: A Comparative Study of Self-Defence Instructors and Courses Operating in Victoria*, unpublished BA Hons Thesis, Dept of Sociology and Women's Studies, La Trobe University, 1991.

Quigley, Toni, *The Lane Cove Survey on Crime and Sexual Assault*, Lane Cove Women's Safety Group, 1984.

Quinn, Kaleghl, *A Woman's Guide to Self-Preservation: Stand Your Ground*, London, Macdonald Optima, 1983.

Ribner, Susan and Chin, Richard, *The Martial Arts*, Harper & Row, New York, 1978.

Russell, Diana E. H., *The Politics of Rape: The Victim's Perspective*, Stein & Day, New York, 1975.

Schnell, Catherine, *Beyond the Dichotomy of Gender: Exploring Women's Physicality*, unpublished BA Thesis, La Trobe University, Melbourne, 1989.

Scutt, Jocelynne, *Women and the Law*, The Law Book Co Ltd, Sydney, 1990.

Sexual Assault Law Reforms in NSW, Department of the Attorney-General & Justice.
Shapcott, David, *Face of the Rapist*, Penguin, Auckland, 1988.
Sheppard, Julia, *Someone Else's Daughter. The Life and Death of Anita Cobby*, Ironbark Press, Sydney, 1991.
St George, Francine, *The Muscle Fitness Book*, Simon & Schuster, Sydney, 1989.
Sydney Rape Crisis Centre, *Surviving Rape*, Redfern Legal Centre, 1990.
White, M., *Going Solo: A Guide for Women Travelling Alone*, STA Travel & Greenhouse, Victoria, 1989.
Wolf, Naomi, *The Beauty Myth*, Vintage, London, 1990.
Women's Advisory Council, *Women and Rape – A Woman's Handbook on Sexual Assault*, Sydney, 1987.
The Women's Co-Ordination Unit, *Information Kit on Sexual Assault*, Sydney, October 1984.
Women's Employment Branch, *Preventing Sexual Harassment in the Workplace: A Guide to Employers*, Department of Labour, Victoria, February 1991.

Videos

All the Difference: Medical Support for Adults Who are Sexually Assaulted, 1990.
Bateman, Py and Lenoyer, Linda, *Peace of Mind*.
Catherine's Story, Dymphna House, NSW Women's Advisory Council, 1990.
Caught Out – Witness under Cross-examination, Health Media, 1990.
Counselling with Interpreters – Sexual Assault Interviews, Health Media, 1988.
'Leave Me Alone: Sexual Harassment Package', Seven Dimensions, Film Australia, 1989.
Lenoyer, Linda, *Alternatives to Fear – A Manual for Instructors*, 1981.
Rape and Older Women – A Guide to Prevention and Protection, US Department of Health and Human Services.
Smith, Bronlyn, *Self-Protection for the Elderly*, Department of Commonwealth Health and Tasmanian Health Department, 1986.

Acknowledgements

I would like to thank my painstaking typist, Barbara Wilson, Carol Middleton (DC Impact), who has sent me copious research material from the USA and has acted as a long-distance sounding board. Ursula Atkinson and Stella Edmundson have been my short-distance sounding boards helping me to arrange my thoughts when they have been addled.

Thanks to C. Moore Hardy for her wonderful photographs and Erna Sonja Lilje for her diagrams. Thanks to Roz Hanratty for locating quotes.

Thanks to my dad for putting boxing gloves on me when I was six and teaching me how to use them.

Thanks to my long-suffering models: Gaye, Barbara, Erna, Ngaio, Kerrie, Felicity, both Peters, Leonardo, Alex, Ivar, Kay, Craig, David, Lyn and Zidia. Thanks also to the YWCA, Sydney, for the use of their premises for some of the photographic shoots.

Last, but not least I would like to thank my very patient editor and publishers, who have been waiting for the birth of this book for a while now. It's been a long, loving, sometimes painful, labour.